The Makeover Manual

The Makeov

er
Manual

From Color Me Beautiful

MARY SPILLANE

MACMILLAN

This book is dedicated to Liz Baker, CMB's Makeover Queen
and my right arm for the past eight years.

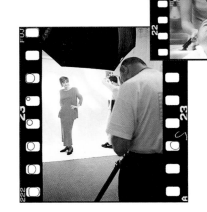

First published 1998 by Macmillan

an imprint of Macmillan Publishers Ltd
25 Eccleston Place, London SW1W 9NF
and Basingstoke

Associated companies throughout the world

ISBN 0 333 71611 6

Text copyright © Mary Spillane 1998
Photographs copyright © Sanders Nicolson 1998,
except where listed on page 186.

The right of Mary Spillane to be identified as the
author of this work has been asserted by her in accordance
with the Copyright, Designs and Patents Act 1988.

9 8 7 6 5 4 3 2 1

A CIP catalogue record for this book is available from
the British Library.

Designed by Macmillan General Books Design Department.
Photographic reproduction by Speedscan, Basildon, Essex.
Printed and bound in Great Britain by Butler & Tanner Ltd,
Frome and London.

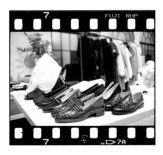

Also by Mary Spillane

The Complete Style Guide
Color Me Beautiful's bible for discovering your best
palette of colours

*Presenting Yourself: A Personal Image Guide
for Women*
A guide to ensure that your business look is
pushing you forward not holding you back.
There is a companion book for men.

Bigger Ideas from Color Me Beautiful
Colour and style advice for the fuller figure

These three titles are published by Piatkus Books

Contents

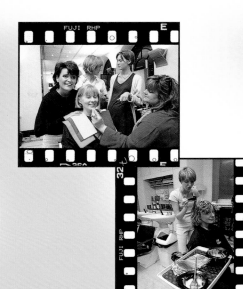

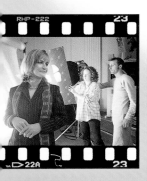
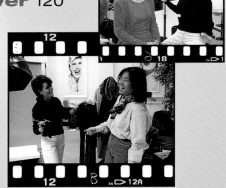

Acknowledgements

Any successful makeover requires a team of talent to create the best possible new look. So has it been for this book, which results from the hard work, cooperation and brilliance of many.

Wella, the hair colour experts, provided technical as well as practical help throughout the preparation of this book. Special thanks go to Jackie Daniels and Technical Director Paul Smith, along with the fantastic team at their London Studios.

Liz Baker and Pippa Newbegin from CMB, along with designer/journalist Tony Glenville, did all the donkey work of selecting and pulling in the clothes to ensure the makeovers were a success. We are grateful to the following PRs and fashion houses for their cooperation: Tiffany & Co., Dickens & Jones, Pallant, Marks and Spencer's, Principles, Liberty, Dorothy Perkins, Favourbrook, Gucci, Evans, Richards, Wallis, Warehouse, Patrick Cox, Coccinelle, Beauchamp Hamling, Boden, Jean Muir, English Eccentrics, Jasper Conran and Mani.

Who could have asked for better models?

My thanks go to this great gang of born-again beauties: Julia Alexander, Janice Daley, Sue Hoare, Emily Hutchings, Jane Levitz, Sue McPherson, Pippa Newbegin, Emma Nicholson, Melissa Ormiston, Rita Ramsey, Sutchinda Rangsi Thompson, Julia Rose, Karen Scott, Ali and Malcolm Wallace, Emma Walmsley, Kate Walmsley, Marie-Louise Windeler, Sarah Wright.

Photographer Sanders Nicolson has the patience of Job and took it in his stride when shots were delayed due to 'sizing difficulties'. Any photographer can make models look terrific. But Sanders made all our makeover candidates look and feel like supermodels.

Hair and Make-up Artists were Sarah Bee, Fiona Corrigan, Diane James, Karen Mason and Dottie Monaghan – each a delight to work with and always teaching us new tricks.

Introduction

Life is long, but it is also too damn short! Why carry on day after day, year after year, feeling less than terrific about yourself? How you look affects how you feel about yourself and influences how others react to you and treat you.

You may be a happy woman, or at least content with who you are and what you have achieved in life so far. Wonderful. This book is for you as much as for women who feel less than fulfilled or not so terrific about themselves – because a truly fulfilled woman is constantly innovating: she changes and grows as the seasons alter and as she meets new people and takes on new responsibilities. She learns, develops skills and becomes more proficient than she thought possible on many levels.

But too often women put their image on hold out of deference to others or to more pressing priorities. 'Once the kids are in school, I can sort myself out.' 'If I get that job, I'll treat myself to a new look.' 'My man likes me the way I am although I hate my size and image.' Living life in neutral is the safe option; with no challenges come no anxieties. But don't you feel more alive when you are challenging yourself, when you learn how to do something better?

Think of the last kick you had from learning something new. Maybe you've mastered a PC, learned to propagate pelargoniums, or taken up tap dancing or salsa. Didn't you feel, in a sense, 'reborn'? Learning and personal development enhance our self-esteem. When we feel good about ourselves, we feel truly alive.

This book is about devoting some time to *you* and your image. It requires you to use your wits and your vision about what you want to look like, and provides you with guidelines for enhancing your current image – or even for revamping yourself totally into a new woman, the next woman of the many in a lifetime that you want to be.

Setting our own continuum

The twenty-first century provides women with many choices. Life is there for the taking and for the making. Our mothers or grandmothers may have had limitations imposed on them, but we do not. There is no charted path scripted at birth or by the age of 21, 40 or 50 that says this is where we are headed, this is what life is going to be. No way. We each need to chart our own path, our own continuum of development. Unforeseen passions become new ways of seeing ourselves, enabling us to reinvent who we are, what we want and how we will give of ourselves.

How we look and how we project ourselves must reflect these changes. As we grow, so too should our image. The young woman who passes her accountancy exams without shedding her student image may linger far longer in that junior post than she needs to. The talented former teacher who wants to try her hand in industry may be written off if she goes to an interview looking like a teacher. The frantic mum who devotes no time to herself (even milliseconds will do!) may find her partner also failing to give her the time and attention she deserves.

There is something self-fulfilling about image: if we look the part we become the part. Treat yourself as a work of art and others will value your creativity. Project the confidence, the warmth and the individuality that you have and others will accept you as being all that and more.

Accentuate the positive

Ask any woman to look in the mirror and tell you what she sees and you will get a laundry list of her shortcomings, every lump and bump. Out of the thousands of women I have worked with over the last fifteen years, it is the rare woman who isn't preoccupied with something: being too short or too tall; having a full bosom or not enough to fill a B cup; full thighs, short legs, no ankles; fine hair, straight hair, curly hair, red hair. An endless catalogue of dissatisfaction.

And yet, unless we unwittingly wear all the wrong things, hardly anyone else notices our problem features.

It's time to dump our obsessions and to work on the whole woman and what she can be. Most problems can be camouflaged or even rectified. For really big challenges, you might need to commit to an exercise regime or submit yourself to the surgeon's knife. Let's not be shy about the possibilities at hand.

Your image is my business

Color Me Beautiful has been the leading personal-image consultancy for real women and men for over fifteen years and has a network that spans the globe. Our colour and style analyses are accurate and straightforward. Millions of women (and men) around the world have been to us for sound advice to take on board and make their own. We do not turn people into something they are not. Each of our sessions is a conversation, a debate or, with some of the strongest characters, a darn good argument. If we were not so effective, people would not return to us again and again for updates, or recommend us so widely to their friends.

Our work has also attracted a lot of media attention, not simply because of the many famous people, leading corporations, politicians and sports personalities who have used us, but because our views are far-reaching and sometimes controversial.

We have had no qualms about telling fashion pundits where to get off with their foolish notions about who should be wearing what and when', just because a coterie of designers and their groupies decided it should be so. We're not anti-fashion at all – we love the innovation and creativity the design world musters each season. It is just that we view fashion from the point of real women who live real lives, and we aim to give them the skills to select the best bits for themselves.

Now the smartest designers – that is, the most 'commercial' ones – have declared that anything goes, any season, so long as it suits the wearer: her colouring, shape, personality and lifestyle. They give us clothes that we love to live in. So, forget worrying about the right hemline for the season and avoid the latest dayglo colour if it makes you look putrid.

How to keep evolving

Women keep asking us for more suggestions, especially on how to recreate themselves or how to break some rules to look and feel like a new person. Hence this book – a guide to making yourself over. You may revisit a few basic strategies on colour and style but you will also be introduced to a

wealth of new ones, and you will be given new ways to tackle shopping and organize your wardrobe, and effective make-up tips.

The first step is to turn to Chapter 1 and to decide how satisfied you are right now with your image and how much you would like to change it.

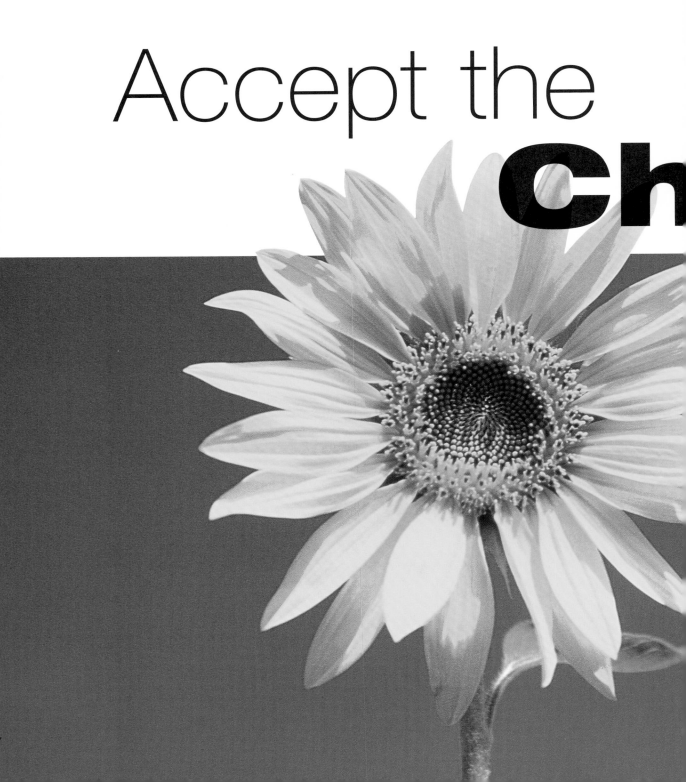

Accept the **Ch**

allenge

Of course you want a new look. Who isn't intrigued to find new ways to express herself? Even if you are Ms Sophisticated with bags of confidence, you are still curious to try new things, to explore new avenues for unlocking more of your personality and true potential.

Whenever there's an opportunity to be 'made over', women queue up. Over the years, we have worked at all sorts of exhibitions, done TV and magazine features and store promotions, and we never cease to come away amazed by the number of women keen as kiddies in a sweet shop to discover a new make-up approach or way to wear their hair. Recently, *Good Housekeeping* magazine in the UK asked us to offer their readers a mini-makeover, and 4000 women wrote, rang and faxed for a place in our studios.

So, none of this dallying about, girl. You know you want a new image and here is the vehicle to get it. The first task is to determine what level of makeover you need. Get a pen and answer **True** or **False** to the following questions.

true *or* false

1   My image has been the same for years.

2   I can't remember the last time I received a compliment.

3   I've longed to look different, better, but don't know where to begin.

4   I look good most days. Looking great, that's less frequent.

5   Make-up hides a multitude of sins.

6   I wish I knew how to play up my features better.

7   I just want to look healthy, not like death warmed up.

8   Clothes can't hide my beastly body.

9   Put me in the hands of a top hair-stylist for an overhaul, please.

10   My body's not perfect, but whose is?

11   The motivation to keep in shape and eat well is lacking.

12   There's little you can do to change my body shape.

13   I have a wardrobe full of clothes but nothing to wear.

14   I often try to copy ideas from friends or magazines, but without success.

15   It's not appropriate for women over 50 to wear fashionable clothes.

16 The real 'me' is seen only at weekends. For work, it's a 'uniform'.

17 I don't look ready for my next career move.

18 Attempts to look sexy or very feminine usually fail.

19 I am no beauty, so why bother?

20 Looking great requires too much time and money.

21 Caring about your appearance is vain.

22 If the Fairy Godmother could wave her magic wand I'd like a perfect bod like a Hollywood star or a supermodel.

23 Shopping is a nightmare.

YOUR SCORES

0 to 5 'True' replies

You are *confident yet challenged* by the possibilities of a new image. You care about the way you look while accepting that you will never be a candidate for the catwalk. But you also know that when you want to you can look pretty damn good.

This book will help you to fine-tune your look and get rid of the baggage that is making you feel stale. If nothing else, it is probably time to clean out the wardrobe and make-up bag.

5 to 10 'True' replies

Complacent but bored best describes your present image. No one is very surprised by how you look but nor have you had the number and kind of compliments you deserve.

Your image is not working for you or against you. So, it's time to shift out of neutral and make some changes. The bets are that you wear lots of the same types of clothes and lack the diversity in your wardrobe to ring the changes. If you haven't experimented with colours, it's time to start. Nothing is more boring than wearing the same combinations all the time.

10 to 15 'True' replies

Dear, oh dear. You are *confused and under-confident*. You've tried a few revamps and failed, mainly because the 'looks' weren't focused on you and the person you want to project. Forget trying to be someone else, or in another body. We can work magic with yours, but first we must work on your self-image.

You have plenty to share with the world – lots of attributes, which start with the woman inside. Try to value those first before worrying about the supposed imperfections. You are letting those worries block our ability to enjoy you and all you have to offer.

You will relate to several of our case studies. Work with them and see which similar approaches you can take. Note the special Clever Camouflage tricks and Morale Boosters: they will reinforce each other.

15 to 20 'True' replies

There is no other way to describe you than *fed up and frantic*. It's been too long since you have felt good about yourself and it's high time to make yourself the priority in your life. Put others on hold for a bit . . . well, at least for long enough to read this book and decide how to take yourself in hand to feel and look better.

I have worked with many terrific women like you, selfless creatures who wake up one day and feel that life is passing them by. You may feel let down by Mother Nature for not blessing you with flawless natural beauty, but simply by being a part of nature you have the potential to be a beauty in your own right.

You'll have a bit more work to do to feel your best. Work that will include some exercise and taking stock of what you eat and drink and how you take care of yourself. If you are prepared to do that, together we can get the look working while you are on the road to feeling better in every respect. Promise you will read the book from cover to cover!

What your answers say about you

1. My image has been the same for years.

    If you have looked the same for many years – same hairstyle, same clothes, same look – you aren't having the fun you could with yourself nor are you exploring all the possibilities for self-expression. Who is holding you back? If it is yourself, be brave and take a step into the unknown. If someone else insists on you staying the same, reassure them (him?) that you will still be the same person inside.

2. I can't remember the last time I received a compliment.

    Compliments should fly in your direction – if not daily, then weekly. By a compliment, I mean anyone who lights up upon seeing you and comments on how well you look. They might not know why you look wonderful but the smile on your face and theirs should be proof that you do.

3. I've longed to look different, better, but don't know where to begin.

    If this is true for you, then you are letting life pass you by. Regardless of budget, age or beauty, you can look different, better, with a little effort.

4. I look good most days. Looking great, that's less frequent.

    Looking great with what you've got should be the objective every day. 'Good enough' means you don't offend but also don't impress. Looking great requires some effort and know-how, not necessarily an unlimited bank account.

5. Make-up hides a multitude of sins.

    Make-up is not for camouflage, it's for enhancing your natural beauty and creating illusions of even greater beauty. See Chapter 7 for how to bring out your best.

6. I wish I knew how to play up my features better.

Let's not wish any longer. Time to learn the tricks of the trade. Use colour to your advantage (Chapter 5) and employ winning style tricks to give you the figure you've always wanted (Chapter 8).

7. I just want to look healthy, not like death warmed up.

Looking healthy should be the basic goal for all women. The colours you wear can make a huge difference (see Chapter 5). If you colour your hair, make sure that it isn't wrong and that it doesn't make you look ill or older (see Chapter 6).

8. Clothes can't hide my beastly body.

The right cut of clothes, fabric and design can hide anything you want. So, whatever bugs you, see Chapter 8 for details of how to disguise it.

9. Put me in the hands of a top hair-stylist for an overhaul, please.

Don't put yourself in the hands of someone to be made over without having your own vision of how you want to look. Bring pictures to convey what you like and get advice about what might be possible for your hair and face shape. Make sure you are shown how to recreate the look before you leave the stylist's.

10. My body's not perfect, but whose is?

So what's perfection? What is considered perfect in one culture, among one age group, during one fashion trend, isn't the same for all. Perfection has nothing to do with image. The best image is the one that reflects the true you and all your potential.

11. The motivation to keep in shape and eat well is lacking.

If you are determined to look and feel terrific you have all the motivation you need to take exercise, eat well and drink in moderation. If you haven't succeeded so far, see all the simple tips in this book for getting into shape and eating well.

12. There's little you can do to change my body shape.

Your basic frame or bone structure, your proportions and your height will stay the same. But through exercise you can build up certain areas and tone down others so as to reduce problem areas. For example, better posture and targeted weight training can enhance the natural shoulder line to help a pear-shaped woman look more balanced. And cosmetic surgery options now make reshaping parts of your body a reality. (See Chapter 4 for details).

13. I have a wardrobe full of clothes but nothing to wear.

If your wardrobe is working against you, time to detox. Pare your clothes down to what you use and love. You will learn the benefits of wardrobe organization in Chapter 9.

14. I often try to copy ideas from friends or magazines, but without success.

You can learn much from being observant about how other women put themselves together. But be sure you stop short of trying to look like them. You are unique – your colouring, shape, proportions and personality are all your own. So, time to discover what works for *you*.

15. It's not appropriate for women over 50 to wear fashionable clothes.

Life and fashion don't end at a certain age. You can and should have fun by looking part of today, regardless of your birth certificate. As an intelligent woman, you know the difference between how you look and how you wear clothes today, and how you were and what you did when you were younger. So use your own good sense, not some dated notion of what's acceptable, to guide you.

16. The real 'me' is seen only at weekends. For work, it's a 'uniform'.

If you aren't projecting the real you in your work clothes, you aren't projecting your best at work. See the advice given to the working women in our makeovers (Chapters 2 and 3).

17. I don't look ready for my next career move.

If you are a career woman you must always look ready for the next move. You have to plant the idea in the minds of the decision-makers that you are the one for the job. The right image can catapult you ahead faster than you realize.

18. Attempts to look sexy or very feminine usually fail.

If you haven't discovered how to look soft, feminine and sexy, it's time you did. Even the most sporty, down-to-earth and busy mum can knock 'em dead. See our makeover in Chapter 2.

19. I am no beauty, so why bother?

Beauty is all relative. So you and I might never be chosen for the catwalk. We should be able to live with that. Just think of how often you have seen a woman at the checkout counter of the supermarket or picking her children up from school who you thought was really beautiful. Indeed, it is all in the eye of the beholder. If there isn't anyone special 'beholding' you at presen, treat yourself like a beauty in your own right and soon there will be someone – if not a few. See Chapter 4 for ideas on 'How to Attract the Man of Your Dreams'.

20. Looking great requires too much time and money.

Can't get off this easily. I have worked with women who buy their clothes from charity shops and look like they just walked off the pages of *Vogue* magazine. A bit of effort takes time and little money. However, how you carry yourself costs nothing but conveys everything. See the section on posture in Chapter 2.

21. Caring about your appearance is vain.

Vanity has nothing to do with wanting to look your best. A good image conveys self-respect and self-esteem. When you treat yourself well, others can only follow.

22. If the Fairy Godmother could wave her magic wand I'd like a perfect bod like a Hollywood star or a supermodel.

You've read about the ups and downs of all those 'beautiful people' featured in *Hello* magazine. So why wallow, dreaming 'if only' dreams. Besides, a diet of lettuce seems a hefty price for thighs the size of a ten-year-old's.

23. Shopping is a nightmare.

Women are supposed to be shopaholics but too many of us find shopping debilitating.

After you learn how to target what is best for you, shopping not only becomes a breeze but also gets more enjoyable. I promise!

Next steps

The makeover you want or need is a personal choice. The following chapters break the makeovers down into three levels: the Beginner, the Intermediate and the Advanced (Chapters 2, 3 and 4).

You can try the quick-and-easy approach with the Beginner Makeover, which requires little in terms of time, effort or investment. Experiment in the morning with our suggestions for revitalizing your hairstyle simply by how you blow it dry. Or wow everyone at teatime by looking as fresh as a daisy thanks to our foolproof make-up tricks that ensure your make-up has lasted all day.

The Intermediate and Advanced makeovers will require some thought and planning. But you are prepared for it because you know it can change your life – well, at least how you feel about yourself and how people respond to you. A career move or new lover could be in the offing.

Chapter 5, The Colour Makeover, is about colour therapy: required reading for all. If you do not know your colour 'season', now is the time to discover it. Or do you know your season already but are feeling a little bored with it? Perhaps it is time to wear the palette differently – or perhaps it's even time to change it. Is this Color Me Beautiful speaking, you might ask? You bet it is. And you'll learn the right directions for changing your natural colouring in Chapter 6.

If you can't cope with your tummy, thighs or bust any longer, jump forthwith to Chapter 8, Your Body Makeover, and learn the art of making the most of your shape. I wish I had a pound for every client who chucked in a tedious diet after learning that she could look slim without losing weight simply by dressing her figure. These tricks are not a licence to throw the rules of good eating to the wind, only a short-cut to looking great while you take steps to get your body in shape, if need be.

You need no better inspiration and proof that our methods work than by reading the experiences of the women who volunteered for the CMB treatment.

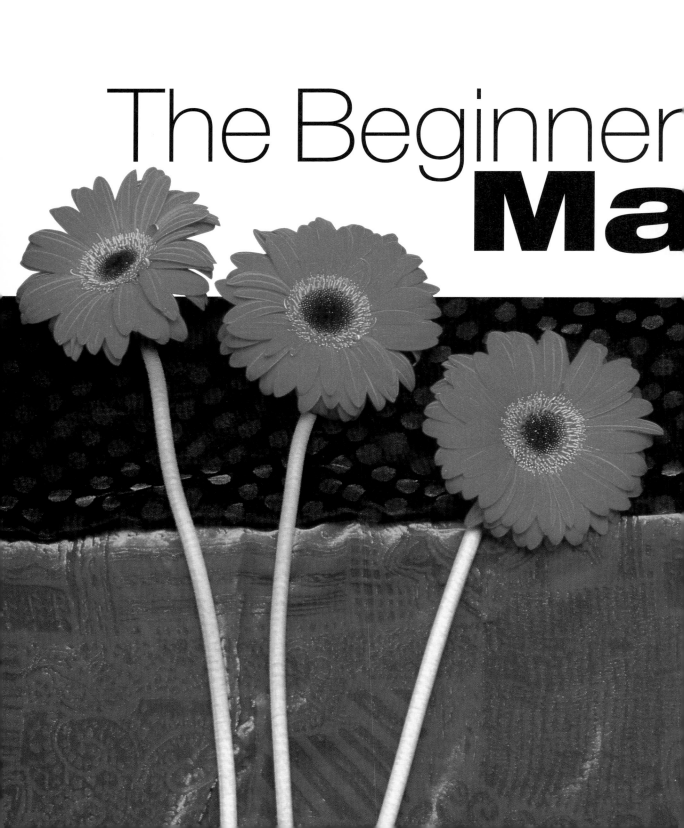

The Beginner
Ma

keover

Okay, okay. Neither you nor your bank account is ready for a total overhaul. But you would like to surprise them at school, the office or at supper tomorrow by looking different. You don't necessarily want to stop traffic but you would like people to notice you and say, 'Hey! What happened last night?'

In this chapter we are going to delve into the possibilities within your own wardrobe and bathroom for looking new and wonderful by tomorrow. Most women have plenty of magic staring them in the face or bursting out of the bathroom cupboard, it's just that they don't know how to use what they have to its full potential or in a new way.

If you have some serious gaps in the fundamentals department you may have to scoot out and purchase a few essentials to pull the new look together.

We'll start with some women who are game to learn a few new approaches to their current wardrobes and beauty routines.

The Career-
Minded Student

JANICE Like many college students, Janice has a packed schedule balancing her studies in business and psychology with a part-time job tending a bar and having a good time. Her current style reflects her creative personality and her desire to be unpredictable. Not all her jeans are so air-conditioned, however!

But the real world looms, with Janice getting ready to hit the job market and to sell both her training and her talents. Her current wardrobe is anything but sensible and she's eager to make the right impression on future employers.

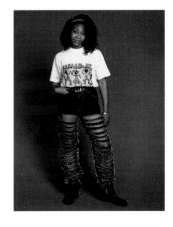

THE RESULT When launching a career, you need to invest in a start-up wardrobe. A bit of judicious planning will ensure that you get your money's worth and have maximum flexibility. This navy blazer is a sure bet for looking smart in just about any environment, and Janice's inverted-triangle body shape looks fabulous, not frumpy, in the blazer's long, lean line. We've opted for soft, fluid stone-coloured trousers to add a touch of sophistication but also to give Janice more versatility than a pair of chinos. She could add a matching stone jacket or top with knits or soft shirts.

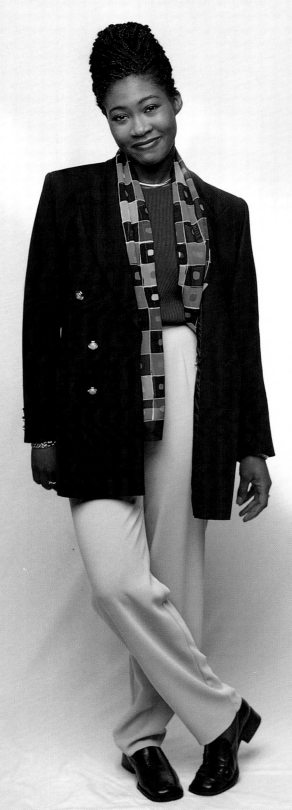

Hair extensions are a great look on Janice but we proved to her that by turning them up into a French twist she can look both different and sophisticated. She looks more business-like and capable and will surely be able to negotiate a better salary than with her fun, carefree hairstyle. Janice has promised to wear her nose ring only on days off, and agrees that when it comes to accessories, less can often prove to be more when your natural good looks are so striking on their own.

STAR TIPS FOR STUDENTS

Be French about it

When on a limited budget, it's smart to follow the French approach to shopping: only buy after you have decided what look you want this season. Comb the fashion mags or visit the chic shops early in the season for some ideas. Also, develop a list of what's missing from your current wardrobe to help you evaluate your choices.

Little pain with plains

Plain fabrics are the most versatile and forgettable. By changing what you wear with them, you can wear them day in and day out without anyone noticing the regularity with which they appear.

Recycle your image

Try second-hand/charity shops in February (spring ranges); May (summer ranges) and September (autumn/winter) for the freshest offerings. Choose shops in the neighbourhoods of the well-heeled for good-quality cast-offs. Best investments are jackets, skirts, trousers and accessories.

Super Mum

ALI Having four children aged six months to nine years means that Ali is lucky if she remembers to wash her own face each morning, although she always looks happy and on top of things and is, no doubt, the envy of many a mother at the school gates.

'I pride myself on being a full-time mother, organizing my children's lives and keeping them all happy. But I would love to know how to pull my look together, and especially what to choose for those rare evenings out with my husband, Malcolm,' explains Ali. With great natural colouring and a terrific, curvy figure (after four kids!), she is sick to death of jeans and T-shirts.

THE RESULT Manic mums have plenty of choice in the new 'jeans' available in fabulous, durable and washable alternatives to denim. These chocolate 'velvet' jeans are smart as well as practical. Likewise with sweaters – no woman need worry about itchy, impractical knit tops with all the

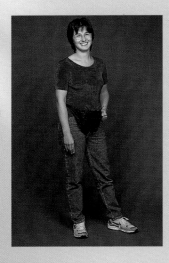

manmade fibres now around, fibres that 'breathe', survive the washer and dryer and look so wonderful. Pull the outfit together with a new-look car coat and super mum will fool everyone that she really is a supermodel.

On the beauty front, Ali needed a few suggestions on how to look and feel as great as she deserves. Very dark hair won't show much change with a semi-permanent rinse, so choose a fairly vibrant shade (quite red in Ali's case) to see just a hint of drama in the daylight. Mums who choose practical short hairstyles should ask themselves if the look is too severe. A few soft wisps at the nape of the neck and/or in the fringe make it sexy as well as easy.

FOR THE EVENING Dress-up choices for busy mothers need to be attractive, able to coordinate with other wardrobe items and capable of lasting a few years. For those precious evenings out with Malcolm, we've suggested one of Ali's 'knock 'em dead' colours (true red) in a washable microfibre with charcoal trousers (not seen). Both pieces can be worn with countless items (the shirt over long or short skirts; the soft, drapy trousers with smart tops, jackets or simple bodysuits). Microfibre is a year-round winning fabric.

As Malcolm is a jeans-and-T-shirt guy, we've given him a terrific sports jacket to smarten up his look for evenings out. Both Ali and Malcolm look perfect for their own idea of a glam night out – not contrived or

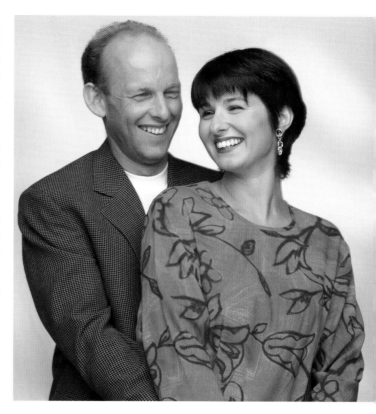

fussy but totally themselves. That's how to do it!

....

STAR TIP FOR MUMS
Colours for kids

Children react to the colours their mums, carers or teachers wear. They respond well to bright colours, especially yellow: you don't need to look like a banana – try a yellow T-shirt or sweatshirt to keep them happy. Avoid greys and beiges, which leave them uneasy, while black and navy can make you look sterner than you want to appear.

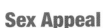

Sex Appeal

Colours for him

Men may respect women in muted tones at the office but they don't necessarily want to have dinner with them. Sludge greens and head-to-toe earth tones leave boys cold as well. To fire the passions try pastels, especially pink. Red can get his blood pumping, but judge when to keep it subtle: sometimes limiting its use to a top, a scarf, fingernails and lips gives the best results.

STAR TIP

Feet first

When you don't know where to begin, start your look from the bottom up. Choose three favourite styles of shoes then build your outfits from them. You will probably want a casual pair, such as boots or loafers; a smart pair, such as court shoes; and a pair of sandals. Ask yourself how well a skirt length or fabric teams with the shoes before you purchase it. Team dressier trousers with smarter shoes, while wearing casual shoes only with your jeans, chinos or leggings.

Sex Appeal

Young parents need to remember to rekindle the flame for each other: it is not just the babies and children that are important in life. Here's how.

- Make regular time for each other. If life is hectic, book a 'date' at least weekly when you get away from work, family and home and just be together.
- Give him the attention he deserves. Actively listen: hold eye contact, lean forward. We all love to feel we are interesting to others and your body language can convince of your attention as much as what you say. If he is boring you to death with the same old stuff, think of open questions you can ask him (that he can't answer yes or no to), such as, 'Where should we explore on our next holiday?' or, 'Who haven't we seen for some time and should get together with?'
- Limit the amount of time you spend discussing tedious household business when out on your 'dates'. Get the leaking tap or the problems with the kids out of the way early, then try to explore broader subjects to get you both animated.
- Don't stay out too late, so that you still have some energy for sex when you get home. Put the moves on him if he's getting lethargic about initiating things. Regular sex is key to staying close as well as keeping young and happy.

Investments You'll
Never Regret

SUTCHINDA Many modern career women have greeted the relaxation in office dress with enthusiasm, particularly for jobs that require freedom of movement or that might call for getting grubby. Artist and book designer Sutchinda opts for comfortable jeans and cotton sweaters or blouses for her daytime 'uniform', as she needs to split her time between meetings, photo shoots or pasting up layouts in her studio. She hastens to point out that 'dressing down' never means being scruffy.

'For me the challenge is those really dressy occasions when other women like to put on party dresses. I feel ridiculous dressed like a doll but I do like to look chic,' she explained.

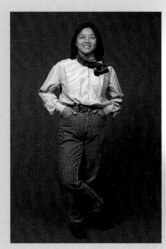

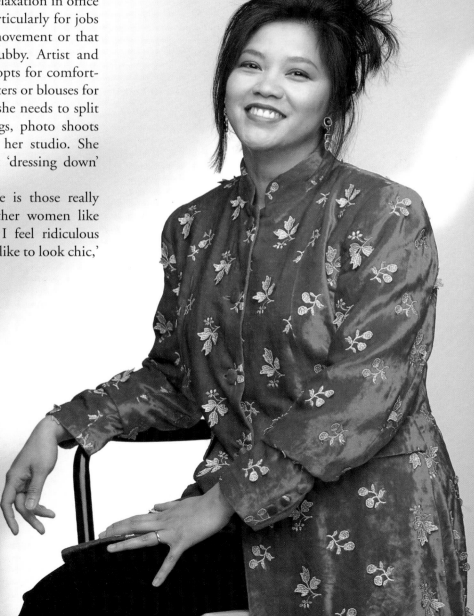

Women like Sutchinda with natural-style personalities need to feel comfortable – day and evening – but require some encouragement when it comes to dressing up. My advice is to invest in a striking top or jacket, in a great colour, that you can wear with trousers or over a simple dress and always turn heads.

THE RESULT Sutchinda was horrified at the price of the jacket. '£500! You can't be serious,' she exclaimed. 'I've never spent that much on clothes.' Calculator to hand, we discussed the return on her investment over the next ten years. And that is being conservative: a jacket like this could be enjoyed for life and then given to your daughter to enjoy as well. I have two such jackets myself, one in embroidered silk for the summer and another in velvet for winter, which I team with skirts, evening pants or jeans, as well as short and long dresses. Not only do they fit the bill but they always make me feel special – the whole point of dressing up!

A beautiful top always draws attention to your face, so Sutchinda needed a lesson in evening make-up to complete the job. Since she wears no make-up at all, only the basics were required to make her dazzle in the evening. She was shocked at first by the red lipstick but when her husband was thrilled with the results she agreed to give it a try in future.

Natural women need only use a simple chopstick to twist their hair up and secure it into place to create a dramatic evening look.

The Clubber
Tries Chic

PIPPA Trendy twenty-somethings soon face the realization that their clubbing gear does not translate to more dressy occasions. When invitations to cocktail and dinner parties or corporate hospitality events start to arrive, you are wise to rethink your dress-up options.

An evening outfit is a serious investment and one you should think long and hard about before making. Pippa was in that dilemma when an invitation came to join her boyfriend and his clients at a black-tie dinner dance. 'I need to look sophisticated and elegant and know that my fun little dresses will let me down,' she explained.

and knowledgeable about your music and who can give you some suggestions about new releases worth trying. Have a listen before you buy – one man's meat is another woman's poison.

Compliment someone else: By making someone else's day you make your own. Always be genuine, never false. If the compliment isn't believable, your eyes and body language will give you away.

Explore your world regularly: Take a different route to work, try a new spot for lunch, go for a walk in a neighbourhood you've always wanted to see. We often think that the great adventure must be further afield and ignore the potential new experiences that are right under our noses. Who knows what natural wonder can be peeked at in someone's garden, or what wonderful person might be shuffling in the book store is just around the corner.

Awaken your senses: Try using drops of essential oils in your bath, or dose a scent ring and place it over a light bulb to allow the therapeutic scent to waft around you. Aromatherapy can help rectify everything from boredom and irritability to a headache and PMS.

Get a dog, cat or rabbit: If you want a living creature in your life that is always happy to see you and wants little more than some love, feeding and exercise, get a pet. But before you do, always consider all the pet's needs as well as your own.

Daydream: Release your creative unconscious into your consciousness. Brilliant ideas as well as solutions to problems may be bubbling quite close to the surface of your mind but unable to get through because you don't allow any time to muse. When the ideas start percolating, sit quietly and allow them to come forth. If your life is hectic, find time and space to let some daydreaming in.

Make a meal of it: How many meals a week are really just refuelling sessions? Try treating yourself to a meal by creating the right ambience, selecting the right dining companion and allowing ample time to make it truly wonderful. Put on music, set a lovely table, light the candles and watch a simple meal turn into a feast.

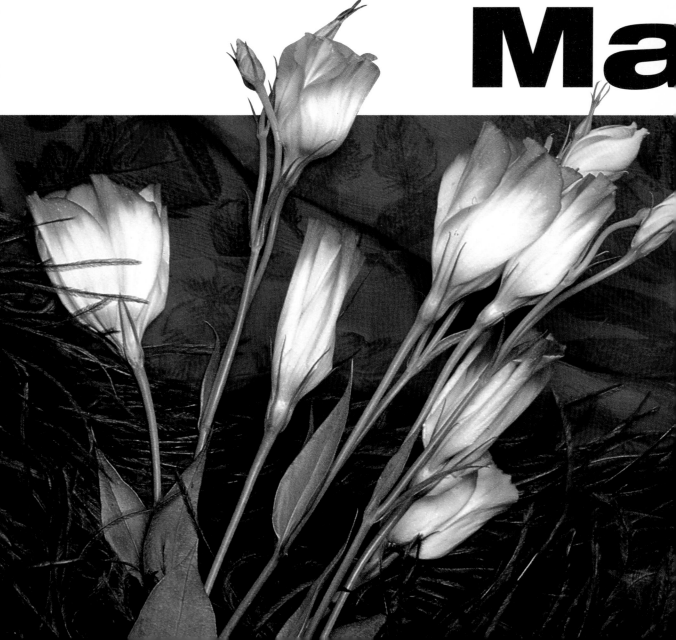

The Intermediate
Ma

ate
keover

You are looking for more than a quick fix to get your image sorted and are keen to learn all the tricks that we image consultants use to teach people how to make the most of themselves.

In this chapter we will take seven women through the process of learning what suits them. You will be able to do the same for yourself by reading more on colour analysis (Chapter 5), make-up (Chapter 7) and body shape (Chapter 8).

A new look often starts with a new hairstyle. Discover how to select the right hairstyle for your face shape, hair texture and personality and never risk getting it wrong again. If you want to be even more experimental and change the colour of your hair, Chapter 6 will tell you how.

It might be time to assess your accessories – clear away the ones you no longer need or want, and then get into the habit of using those you do. Add the finishing touch with a cleverly tied scarf: some of the best but easiest and most effective ways are illustrated on page 53.

Find out how to maximize your smile by caring for your teeth and improving their condition with the tips on dental hygiene. (But for taking modern dentistry to its limits, see the next chapter, The Advanced Makeover.)

Seeing is Believing

JULIE When a super secretary gets picked for the top office to become Personal Assistant to the Chief Executive, her wardrobe requires a rethink. Power suits can be ageing and might be perceived by colleagues as dressing above your position. Sharp suits would be an unlikely choice for a young woman like Julie who is friendly and fun as well as incredibly capable. She wants to present a polished, efficient welcome to all her boss's important visitors but also to project no-nonsense authority when having to sort out problems.

Julie looks smart enough as a secretary and knows that an extra layer like a simple waistcoat can add panache to a skirt and blouse. But the trendy, clumpy shoes make the look less professional and elegant – a mistake young working women often make. The overall look is junior secretary, not Executive PA.

THE RESULT When you need to smarten up, try a fresh hairstyle to bring yourself up to date. This layered, feathered style is both fun and flattering on Julie. We've combed in very gentle streaks to give her hair a sun-kissed glow – a good first step for the colour-timid. (For more tips on your hairstyle see page 54.) With a lesson in make-up grooming, Julie looks more polished.

Simple shift dresses look elegant for doing business during the day or evening, and when teamed with a prettily coloured jacket help Julie stand out from the sea of neutral power suits that the company's female managers make.

Julie was interested to learn more about colours but winced at first sight of this burnt-orange outfit, our suggested alternative for more relaxed, outdoor corporate hospitality events, such as a day at the races, or a golf competition or tennis tournament. Easy knits are the perfect choice for busy working women who need to take a quick change to the office for a mid-day transformation. Julie was so taken by the look, as well as the reasonable value of this High Street choice, that she bought the outfit for herself.

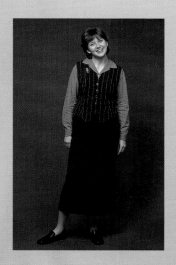

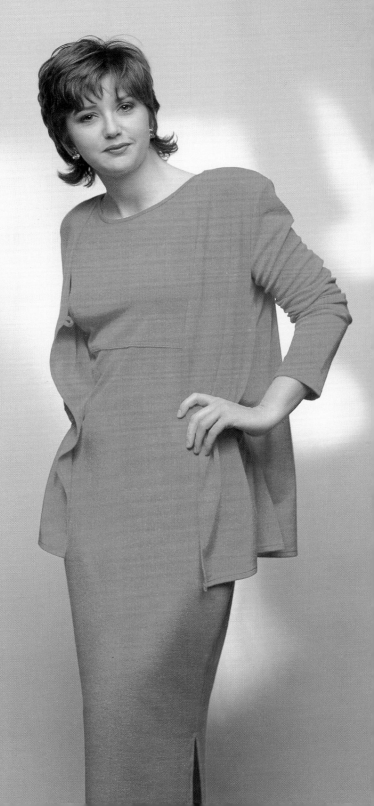

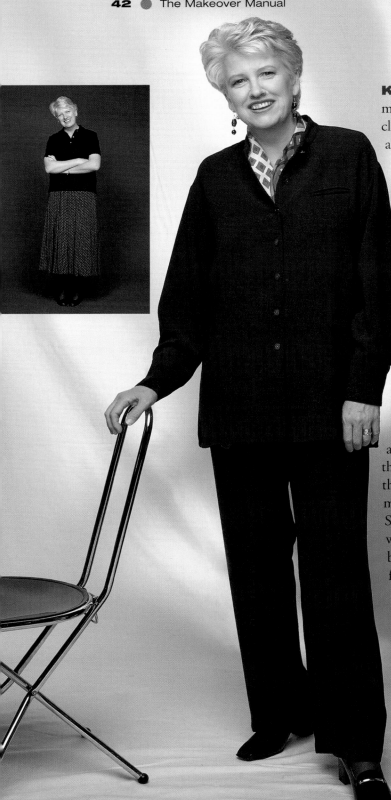

KATE You would never know that Julie's mother Kate had been working round the clock for thirty-six hours. When I asked about her normal work schedule, she replied simply 'full-time and variable': just what you would expect from a committed midwife on call to help women give birth at home. Needless to say, her practical day-to-day look is T-shirt, leggings and bare feet – 'We encourage water babies,' she explains.

When she is out promoting home births to women's groups, a blouse and skirt are the usual choice. 'I think this is appropriate, but my guess is you might consider it a bit boring,' she said with a pleading tone that suggested please say it's okay.

I so enjoy working with women like Kate – lovely, interesting women worried about how to dress their 'age'. My answer is that you are part of this age and as we hit the new millennium you should look as much a part of the future as your daughter. Sure, you will do it differently. But let's not write off having fun with fashion just because you have white hair or a mid-life figure.

THE RESULT Kate was thrilled with this relaxed 'suit' – a shirt/jacket and easy trousers. The longer top takes the emphasis off her tummy ('at 50 it just appeared'), helping her look long, lean and two sizes smaller. This particular navy has plum undertones and is more flattering than very dark, inky versions of navy. With her cool, soft colouring, Kate will look, lovely in many shades of purple, from the sheerest lilacs and violets through to plum and aubergine.

Like mother, like daughter?
A softer figure like Kate's will always look feminine as well as practical in trouser suits that aren't overly tailored and drape easily over her shape. In a more structured jacket and heavier fabrics Kate would look heavy as well as uncomfortable. Also, as one ages very tailored styles, especially in trouser suits, can appear severe, even downright 'butch'. So employ a few feminine touches when wearing these sensible outfits by styling your hair, applying make-up and adding a dash of perfume.

Office Makeover
Essentials

Every working woman needs to dress for comfort as well as impact. To perform your own makeover in the office on a day that something important and unexpected crops up, have the following gear to hand. If you work in an office with other women, see which items you can share (e.g. a hairdryer, magnifying mirror, cotton wool).

Make-up essentials
> powder
> lip pencil and lipstick
> mascara
> cotton wool and tissues

Before any important meeting, check your powder and lipstick. If you did without make-up this morning (shame!), add a brushing of mascara.

Hair essentials
> styling spray
> styling brush
> hair dryer

If you got caught in the rain, or meant to do your hair this morning, spray underneath your hair then turn your head upside down and use the dryer for 2 to 3 minutes on the roots alone. Lift your head and style. Fuller and fluffier, you will frame your face more effectively and look more polished.

Grooming essentials

spare tights (natural, sheer
black/navy)

emery board

clear nail varnish and remover

cuticle and hand cream

Give your hands a 3-minute makeover before a big meeting by quickly filing rough tips and giving a quick clear varnish. When the varnish is dry, use cuticle and hand cream. Try never to attend an important meeting with chipped or dirty nails.

Style essentials

jacket

earrings

good pen

papers organized

Always put on a jacket before an important meeting. If you will be presenting standing up, button your jacket to keep the attention on your face (and away from your bust). Earrings will help you look smart and polished. Arriving with your papers organized in a file and a smart (rather than disposable) pen shows that you are a woman ready for anything.

Office Options

Jackets: When in doubt, don the armour. Test the different reception you receive with and without a jacket. You'll be amazed how much more seriously you are taken with your 'shield'.

Skirts: Opt for designs that can run, squat, get in and out of cars, and last in front of the computer for hours on end. If yours let you down by riding up or developing horizontal stretch marks, it's time to choose a different size, fabric and cut.

Belts: Finish off your skirts and trousers with a good belt to look pulled together in every sense. Choose plain calf leather or styles with minimal design for greatest polish.

Tailored or trendy: It's not up to you but to the company to guide on this. Look too unlike the corporate image and plan on a lonely, possibly short, stint in your current post.

Career and Image
Makeover

KAREN At 39 Karen gave up trying to superwoman, handling a marketing job while trying to raise two young children. Now she's happy being super mum, but has also turned her hand to interior design. She started by revamping her own home and now plans to market her talents to others. 'Needless to say, my own image has been on hold for a while. I'd love to know how to repackage myself, especially now that I don't have to wear suits every day.'

Karen describes her present image as the 'desperately confused mum'. Six months ago, she chopped off her waist-length hair and had a disappointing perm.

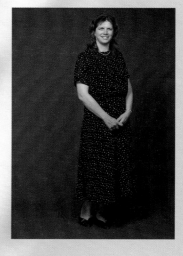

With the dregs of the perm and a growing-out hairstyle she's in need of fresh advice on both colour and cut. She knows she should bother with make-up and agrees that she needs brightening up but is terrified to wear a lot of colour on her face. Our job is to prove that the right colours won't look garish but make more of her lovely features and natural good looks.

Karen's classic dress belies her natural, creative personality. Her frame is large and simply looks larger in a flimsy, delicately patterned fabric. Dresses are too fussy and prim for any woman likely to play on the

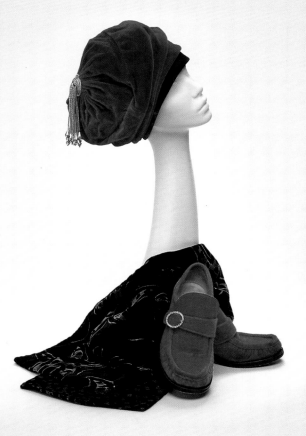

floor with the kids one minute and dip a brush into a pot of paint the next. Importantly, we also want Karen's image to sell her new potential as an interior decorator. So a new look is required.

THE RESULT Medium-depth brown hair has many exciting options for colouring, such as damson or rich auburn. By deepening the hair colour, Karen's bit of grey blends away perfectly, while the lustre becomes richer thanks to the benefits of a semi-permanent colour conditioning.

Bigger women need to be wary of cropped hairstyles that can be out of scale with their frames. So we tapered Karen's hair with soft layers but added fullness and softness by styling with a large brush. Her make-up uses deep, rich colours of plum and grey which complement her cool, clear colouring better than her own light, pastel tones.

We chose a fabulous purple top with a self-pattern mixing velvet and a transparent chiffon, great for Karen to look both creative and feminine. A superb fitting pair of black trousers is a must in most wardrobes, and these trousers have an ample dose of Lycra to make them comfortable as well as smart.

Karen's new look gave her a real boost and the confidence to be both more colourful and bolder with her style.

Top Ten Tips
for Mums Who Don't Want to Look Mumsy

To be effective and get the credit they deserve for labours done outside headquarters, home-based career women need to take special steps to look part of the scene when opportunities arise to mingle with office-bound colleagues. I've seen these gems arrive for meetings in a frenzied state, breathless with some domestic nightmare, unmade-up with hair sorely in need of attention and totally unaware of what they are wearing.

Once a management consultant came to a meeting in a floral dress and scuffed driving shoes as she was too preoccupied to remember to put the right ones on. The dress was pretty, definitely mumsy, but not the right image in which to deliver a project review.

HERE ARE MY TOP TEN TIPS FOR MUMS WHO DON'T WANT TO LOOK MUMSY:

✦ Aim for a 'suited' effect when pulling separates together. Always wear a jacket layer, even if it is a substantial blouse (e.g. in summertime) over a dress.

✦ Avoid florals: they scream either 'tea party' or 'mummy'.

✦ Pull longer hair back into a smart clip. Short hair should be styled to frame the face, not just combed neatly.

✦ Wear make-up – don't cheat with just lipstick and powder (all mums do that to go to the supermarket).

✦ Wear earrings for meetings to show you mean business.

✦ Avoid carrying shopping bags to business meetings. Invest in a smart leather 'shopper' that can hold papers, a loaf of bread and pint of milk without anyone knowing.

✦ Fine yet hard-wearing hosiery and shoes will convey that you are doing well as a freelance. Polish shoes regularly if you also use them to scoot out to the garden to rescue clothes from the washing line.

✦ Wear clothes that fit you now, not ones that once did.

✦ Smell smart, not like disinfectant.

✦ Aim to arrive for meetings 10 minutes early to calm down and get on top of the business at hand.

A Cross-Cultural
Makeover

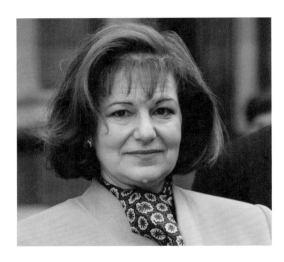

EMMA NICHOLSON Liberal Democrat peer, human rights advocate and aspiring Member of the European Parliament, Emma has always been considered one of the smartest, most polished women in the British political arena.

Emma's classic, elegant style is best described as quintessentially English. Her well-tailored clothes have had to work as hard as she does and take her through a demanding schedule of briefings, meetings and speeches from morning till night. It is a challenge for all female MPs that they need to look terrific giving a speech at midnight in the House that will be seen by the nation on prime-time television the next

day. 'Hence, I keep my hairstyle simple and am sure to have make-up with me at all times,' she explains.

On resigning as an MP and to enhance her new role in the House of Lords, Emma wanted advice on how to fine-tune her look. What should she do differently as she ages but still expects to be in the limelight? As with many high-profile women, Emma has mastered the basics of looking her best and prides herself on knowing not only what she likes but also what suits her. A recent convert to trouser suits, after years in proper, skirted power suits, Emma wants help with selecting styles and fabrics that transfer from day to evening better than her linen and woollen ones, which look too 'daytime' at a cocktail reception. With her ambitions now firmly on the European parliament, Emma also wants clothes that look both modern and more international than some very traditional British styles succeed in doing.

THE RESULT Emma's hairstyle was modified with a softer, more modern look and benefited from a new approach with colouring. Currently she is using a tint a few shades deeper than her natural colour, the effect of which is slightly harsh on her skin tone. For

any woman like Emma with striking natural colouring who wants to keep the grey
at bay it is better to lighten the effect
around the face and keep the depth back. A
few highlighted sections in warm gold,
beige and copper were much more becoming on Emma's skin. Then we used an
auburn semi-permanent rinse to give a
warmer shine to her basic tint.

Emma wanted another black trouser
suit to take her from day to evening. 'I
know black is a bit strong on me but it is so
useful.' As image consultants we deal with
realities such as this and aim to show women
how to wear colours that might not be their
absolute best. With soft, warm colouring,
Emma needs to soften the impact of black
with a warm-tone blouse and scarf.

This suit in draped jersey is not only
the most comfortable option for a day-to-
evening transition but less likely to date
than a tailored, fitted style. When you are
looking for something classic, be sure it's
modern. Some supposed 'classics' have been
around so many years that although they
might be new they look 'old' because the
style and fabric are so dated.

When women begin to notice that
their necks are starting to show their age,
they often try to hide the lines
with a scarf. Emma is more
flattered by having an
open neck and a
softer drape to her
scarves. When you
frame your face with
the right colours and
styles people don't focus
on minor imperfections,
just on you.

Accessories
Makeover

If your look isn't quite 'pulled together', maybe it's because your accessories are letting you down. Indeed, your shoes, handbag, watch, jewellery and all the extra bits convey subtle but important messages about your personality and lifestyle. Do your accessories complement each other and you, or do they fight for attention?

It's a cinch to recognize when accessories are wrong for an outfit: the 'cleverly tied' scarf, the gold-embossed logo belt or the shoes that wear the woman. Deciding what is right for a particular outfit is subjective and must take into account both the personality of the wearer and the occasion. You know which earrings are your favourites, and why and how a particular belt or bag seems to work with everything. You want the same confidence and versatility in all of your accessories and so you need to know which additional items are the real treats to bring out when you want either to dazzle or to shock.

The right to retire

As with the rest of your wardrobe, every now and then your accessories deserve a good clear out and store-away for your daughters or for fancy-dress parties. For accessories you no longer want to keep, consider handing them over to a church or charity jumble sale.

Be ruthless about the future wearability of everything you keep. Scarves can last for years, but if the fabric is inferior and the pattern dated why have them clutter your drawers any longer? Maybe you've finally decided, after years of trying to be clever with scarves or belts, that you aren't a scarf or belt person. If your neck is short, scarves will make you look podgy. If you have a wide waist, belts will only accentuate it. So see if you need every category of accessory or whether you should finally retire one for good.

If any piece of jewellery is nicked or tarnished, ask yourself if it can be repaired (for less than the value of the piece itself). If not, retire it.

But is it YOU?

Your accessories should express the woman inside. Maybe after years of wearing classic button earrings, you find yourself hating them. Perhaps you feel much more imaginative and creative now than you have before. Boring earrings on a creative woman look out of sync with her own personal flair.

Some jewellery has great sentimental value but not so much versatility, and you need to know how to wear it. A family cameo or locket is a good example. Try wearing traditional pieces on plain fabrics such as a simple shift dress or twinset rather than on a business suit or printed fabric.

If your accessories are letting your image down and saying other things about you than you want said, then get hunting for pieces that express your personality. Shopping for clothes can become just a functional activity, especially when looking for replacement items, but shopping for accessories can be a real treat. You don't have to settle for anything less than wonderful (at the right price, of course) and you should seek out sources that will provide you with bits that aren't seen every day on everyone else.

Essential Accessories

Watch: Get one that can do for day and evening, so avoid plastic. Scale the size to your bone structure: delicate if fine-boned, substantial if big-boned.

Necklaces: Find a winner made of pearl, gold, silver, or gold and silver that you can wear every day without thinking about it. It should be appropriate with a T-shirt or a business suit, so not too small or too large. After your daytime basic, opt for additional stones, beads or metal in varying lengths to give you the widest possible choice for your current lifestyle. If you rarely go to glittering events, borrow diamanté (or, if lucky, diamonds!) and spend your money only on a chain or string of crafted beads that you will wear several times a month.

Earrings: If most of your earrings are alike, think of a particular outfit to which you find it hard to match your earrings. Then start to expand your range by matching this outfit with earrings. Opt for variety in metal and design but follow your instincts and resist too much experimentation. Trendy plastic earrings are probably going too far. Choose more timeless (but not boring) designs.

Rings: Nothing destroys the impact of a lovely ring better than being cluttered with too many others. If you love wearing more than one ring on each hand, make sure the metals and designs don't fight each other. Rings draw attention to hands so ensure that yours are worth the look. Keep your nails manicured (not necessarily varnished) and your hands protected daily with cream.

Bracelets: There are ring freaks and bracelet freaks and, yes, sometimes they are one and the same person. A funky girl who loves an armload of jangling bangles has learned to live with the clanging and is probably unaware of the effect she has on everyone else's nervous system. In business, if your bracelets make a noise, they are inappropriate. Limit to one per wrist or, better, wear only on the arm you don't use for writing so that the bracelet will not clang every time you put pen to paper (particularly distracting for others in meetings).

Wood and plastic should be reserved for summertime and picnics.

Belts: If you wear skirts and trousers with belt loops it is nice to complete the outfit with a belt. Don't expect one belt to look terrific with both jeans and business suit. A clumpy, braided belt with a fine dress or business suit doesn't work, and jeans lose their panache with a patent leather or chain belt.

If you have a well-defined or long waist, you can wear a variety of belts. If your waist is wide, wear a belt to tone in (not contrast) with the colour of your skirts and trousers. If you are short-waisted, avoid the loops on waistbands and wear your belt slung over the hips on top of a blouse or top. Ideally, shop for a belt while wearing the clothes for which it is intended.

If you like them, remember you only ever need one chain belt.

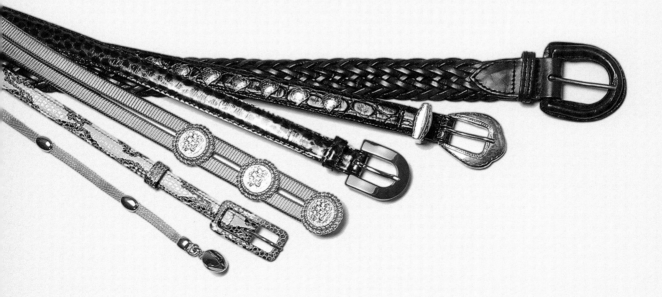

Scarves

If you haven't discovered the wonders of scarves, it is time you did. Probably the easiest and cheapest way to change the look of a whole outfit is with a scarf, whether it be a simple pocket handkerchief or a smart cravat at the neck, or a larger oblong of colour and texture to double up as a wrap.

Let a patterned scarf be the centre of attention in an outfit. Provide the right backdrop of minimal fuss, colour and fabric contrasts, and no other pattern unless almost indistinguishable.

Square scarves

Squares provide many, many possibilities for filling a neckline (don't forget they can act as a belt too). Here are just a few of the easiest ones to master.

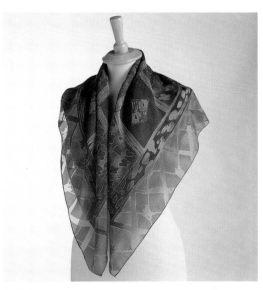

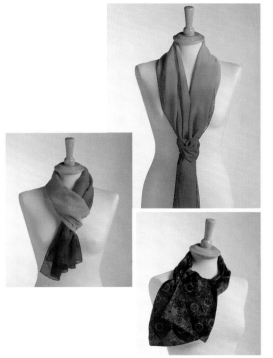

Oblong scarves

Oblongs are the best alternative if you want to have minimal fuss with maximum impact. They can be worn inside a jacket or wrapped around the neck or shoulders for drama. A long, lean oblong creates a slimming effect: good for fuller figures. If petite, be careful not to wear the very long versions or you'll look like you are wearing a blanket.

The Makeover for
Your Hairstyle

A new hairstyle transforms your look more quickly than anything. That's why it's important to see if your hairstyle and colour are making the most of your features and personality.

Three factors are vital in choosing a hairstyle: your face shape, hair texture and personality.

Face shape

Sadly, many hairdressers don't take into account the shape of your face from the front and side before giving you a new look. A good stylist is an artist who knows how to flatter your features. But too often you are given a great new style that is completely wrong for you.

Unless you have an oval face with fairly balanced proportions and easy features, the best advice is not to repeat the shape of your face but to complement it. A round hairstyle on a round face is not interesting or flattering. A sharp angular bob on a square face not only makes the face more square but looks severe.

To determine your face shape, first scrape your hair back in a headband or clips. For fun, put some dots with a bit of foundation, lipstick or concealer on a few key points on your face to help you see the outline better: two dots above the eyes near the hairline; a dot on each temple; two dots on the widest point on the face: forehead, cheeks or jaw; and two dots on the chin line directly below the outer edge of the eyes. Imagine you could connect up the dots. Now select the shape face that most closely matches yours.

OVAL FACE The face is evenly proportioned with the forehead as the widest point (only slightly). Your only limits on style selection come down to the texture of your hair and your personality.

ROUND FACE The fullest point will be the cheeks. The overall effect is short and wide. To balance your features, choose styles that add height and length. Avoid fullness on the sides and centre partings. A long sleek style can dramatically play up your features.

HEART FACE The forehead is the widest part and the chin is very narrow. To minimize the impact of your forehead, use a side parting or consider a fringe that is brushed sideways to create an angle that 'cuts' the forehead by a third or half. Balance at the chin with soft wisps or curls that fall softly and add volume.

PEAR FACE The widest point is the jawline, with the forehead narrower. Add volume at the top with layers in a short, angled crop or keep it long and sleek but with soft layers in a fringe (brushed back or to the side) and around the top of your face. Keep some of the forehead in view.

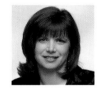

SQUARE FACE The same width at temples and jawline. Like the oval, the face is short and wide but on a square face the features are more pronounced. Choose styles that add height and minimize width. Soft layering on top is good, while soft wisps or curls can soften the 'edges'. If the face is quite wide, keep hair behind your ears to reduce volume on the sides, while some length at the neck will soften your jawline.

RECTANGULAR FACE The forehead, temples and jaw are equally wide and the face is distinctly long and narrow. The goal is to minimize height and length and to create some fullness. A fringe is the easiest way to 'shorten' your face, with a short, full bob completing the job of creating balance.

DIAMOND FACE The cheekbones are the widest point, with the forehead and jaw narrow. Your objectives are threefold: accentuate your lovely cheeks, keep the forehead light, and soften at the jawline. So no top-heavy styles or dense straight fringes. Try layered, brushed-back or feathered styles that show off your features from the front and side. Longer styles are fine, as well as medium lengths that layer into the jaw and neckline.

Hair texture

The natural texture of your hair is down to your genes. However, a variety of other factors contribute to making it better or worse: hormonal changes, climatic circumstances, pollution and humidity.

When you look for a new style, find out how much daily effort is required to achieve the style with your hair texture. Even lank and lifeless hair, with the right shampoo and styling products, can look full and bouncy. If you haven't had success to date in getting what you want from your hair, it's time to see a specialist. Seek out the most expert hairdresser in your area or travel to the nearest city where there are hairdressers with up-to-date know-how.

When searching for a new hairdresser, start by asking advice from friends whose styles you like. Ask your most experimental pals who they use and why. While you might not be as daring as they are, if their styles are effective they are probably seeing a talented stylist. If your area isn't a hotbed of hairdressing talent, be prepared to travel for some sage styling. Read regional newspapers and magazines and note which salons are credited in the makeovers. Don't hesitate to ring up the beauty editor and ask her advice on someone good.

Bring along pictures from magazines of 'looks' that you'd like to try, and ask how achievable they might be for you (considering your own hair and how much effort you are willing to put in to create the effect). Get advice on the myriad selection of helpful styling products or treatments like perms that could transform the natural condition and performance of your hair quite dramatically.

Don't let any stylist start snipping until you feel confident s/he understands your expectations. The best salons will even grant you a free consultation before committing to an appointment. You should have a complete consultation with your stylist prior to shampooing to be able to discuss your hair in its natural state. If you are in any doubt about their skills or sensitivity to your wants don't hesitate to say that you have changed your mind and leave. A moment's embarrassment might save you a month in hiding.

For any chronic scalp or hair problems consult a trichologist, who will restore the health of your hair from within by recommending vitamin supplements and counselling you on your diet, as well as from without by providing specific treatments for your condition.

Personality

The final factor to take into account in selecting your best hairstyle, along with face shape and hair texture, is your own personality. Adapt the recommendations for your face shape to achieve the look that suits you.

For example, let's say your hair is naturally curly and presently shoulder length, but you would like to look more dramatic, a bit sharper. The texture of your hair can't be sharpened but by selecting an angular cut and using a gloss or gel to tame your curls you can, indeed, look very sleek.

Another challenge is for a woman with sharp features, say a strong jawline, and straight hair who wants to look softer and more romantic. She can do so by cutting her hair in softer layers; getting an acid (soft) perm to add volume and wave, and using pretty clips or headbands to add a feminine touch.

So take all three factors into account when selecting a new hairstyle: complement, don't repeat, your face shape; make the most of your natural hair texture; and project your personality. If your current hairdresser can't help you, it's time to shop around for someone who is both more knowledgeable and sympathetic.

The Makeover for Your Smile:
Beautiful Teeth

Sadly, the teeth get short-changed in the daily beauty regime. A few hectic minutes of brushing is usually all the attention they receive but the teeth are on view full-time, big-time every day and can ruin all your other beauty efforts if you don't do the basics to keep them in good health and condition.

The right tools

Chances are that you are more particular about the kind of brush you use to style your hair and about your best kind of shampoo than you are about your toothbrush and paste.

The right brush can not only encourage you to brush longer (ideally for 2 to 3 minutes twice a day), but also improve the health of your gums, so important to sustaining your teeth in the long run.

Your toothbrush: The best investment you can ever make is in an electric toothbrush. Not only do these small heads with their circular movements clean the teeth and gums more effectively than a standard toothbrush can, but they also encourage you to brush for longer (most have a flashing light to signify when you have finished). You feel as though you have had your teeth cleaned professionally every day, and the dentist will confirm the improvement in the health of your mouth at the next visit.

Toothpaste: Choose a toothpaste that whitens, prevents cavities and freshens the breath. Check the ingredients, or ask your dentist what s/he recommends. You probably need something that is effective on everyday stains from tea, coffee, red wine, smoking and fruit juices.

Flossing: Critical to your oral hygiene is to floss daily to remove food that can build up between teeth and gums and cause disease, cavities and bad breath. Have floss packs handy everywhere so you are bound to pick one up and do it when you have a spare minute. I confess to having floss in my car to make the best use of a traffic jam!

Check-Ups: Find a convenient hygienist and commit to going two or three times a year to scrape away surface stains and plaque – key to preventing more serious problems. Tartar build-up is the source of discoloration: its rough surface attracts plaque, which absorbs stains. Make sure the hygienist uses a 'blaster' before polishing – a gun that shoots a salty powder to treat stains. You'll have a refreshing sensation afterwards.

Whitening: For pearly-white teeth like you see on American TV you have to travel to the USA for a bleaching treatment or bleach mould (using peroxide): they are banned in the European Union (rats developed cancer after being injected with rather inordinate amounts of the stuff). But the pressure is on for an alternative treatment to be found.

To reduce the staining effects of tea and red wine, brush once a week with baking soda used directly on the brush. Don't do it more frequently or it will, eventually, remove your tooth enamel.

Corrective dental treatments

Any woman of any age should consider the array of corrective measures that are available to sort out discoloured, cracked and crooked teeth. Bad teeth do more to ruin a woman's natural beauty than anything. A beautifully made-up face won't hide bad teeth. Sure, corrective or 'cosmetic' dental treatments cost money – okay, a small fortune. But I have seen women and men forgo a new car, a holiday and even get a bank loan to sort out their teeth. The result is a tremendous boost to self-confidence. For more on this, see the next chapter.

MORALE BOOSTER

Smile! Tomorrow will be different, better, if you face the world with a smile. If you need convincing, the latest research confirms that smiles and laughter release the super antibody immunoglobulin A, which boosts the immune system. So they are good for your health as well as your image. Try speaking to people with a smile (when appropriate) and watch them mirror that smile straight back. Every face is more beautiful when it is smiling.

Office Options

Casual days: These can be nightmares, especially for chief executives and human resource managers. You work hard so your clothes should be comfortable, but not so comfy that you look like you're off to a picnic. Select quality casuals, in the right fabric for the time of year, and add a few accessories for panache. Always – but always – have a jacket at the ready for an important session with a client or the boss.

Nerves: If you are nervous about a looming presentation or confrontation, get away from the fray (preferably outdoors) and walk briskly for 5 to 10 minutes. Imagine yourself doing brilliantly and getting the right reactions from the audience. A bit of adrenaline management and positive thinking can work wonders.

Presenting your best: You need a look that keeps the attention on your face. Opt for toning plain colours from the waist down with a knock-'em-dead top, but beware of 'interesting' accessories that distract from you, and always button your jacket so that your assets don't outshine your performance.

Cut the clutter: Ask yourself what it is absolutely vital to bring to a meeting and house it in something simple and functional. Don't arrive with multiple bags, parcels and files: a cluttered arrival symbolizes muddled thinking.

Classic court shoes: In navy or black, these are a wardrobe basic for all working women. When in doubt, these finish off a classic suit best of all.

Attaché: Be it a leather shopper/tote, a sleek briefcase or an envelope attaché, it should project serious business to all and sundry. Avoid unnecessary bulk or anything that could take you and your wardrobe away for the weekend. Try to compartmentalize key items for easy access.

Shackets: Shirts worn as jackets are ideal for summertime, especially in offices with pathetic excuses for air-conditioning. Select a blouse of substantial weight, quality and construction, and wear it over a light T-shirt or camisole to keep you cool while you look the business.

Out of Uniform

RITA Women who work in a uniform are blessed with being able to roll out of bed in the morning without struggling to coordinate anything. You might like, hate or be indifferent about the colour and style of it, but at least a uniform takes away that daily hassle of 'What the heck am I going to wear?'

Rita wants to develop her casual look. She's got the relaxed, stay-at-home stuff sorted but she wants help in figuring out what 'smart casual' might be for her. She also wants some help with her hair. Her way of dealing with her fine hair is to twist it up and pin it together. 'I've given up trying to get it into some sort of style,' she sighed. 'It's fruitless – in no time it is drooping around my face.'

Fine hair requires three things: 1) a great cut; 2) a light shampoo; and 3) the right styling spray. Wispy hair can look very trendy if your stylist knows how to create movement and shape. Rita, and women like her, should use pure shampoos designed for fine hair or baby shampoo. Plus: use only a micro amount of conditioner, if any at all. A fine styling spray used on the roots makes styling a cinch and creates welcome volume. Sprays are preferable to sticky gels or heavier mousse formulations.

THE RESULT Knits can be both comfortable and smart. When you see a group of knitted separates, get two or three pieces, at least, from the same collection to give yourself endless possibilities. Along with this great top and skirt, Rita picked up a terrific pair of coordinating trousers and a long knit jacket. All she might need is a scarf, another body or a T-shirt and a pair of boots and she could be off for the weekend.

Mid-lifers like Rita sometimes fret about revisiting a style they wore years ago. 'Don't I look frumpy in a long skirt?' she asked. Indeed not! If a woman chooses modern fabrics and cuts that suit her, she looks terrific at any age.

And with a totally new approach to her make-up, Rita couldn't stop giggling at the result. 'Is that really me? I never thought I could look this good!'

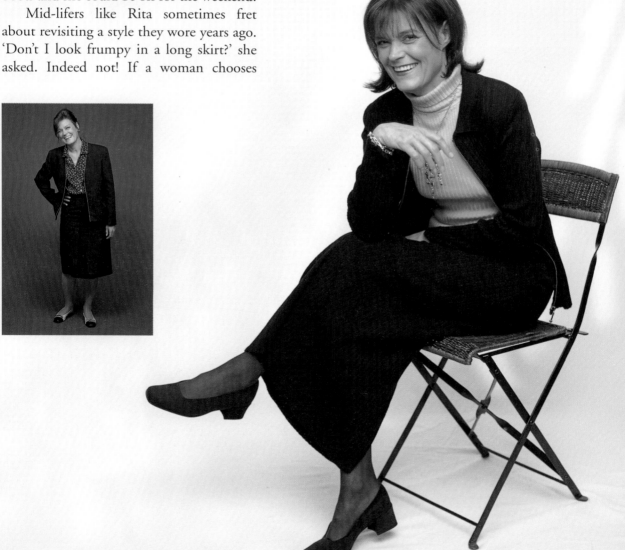

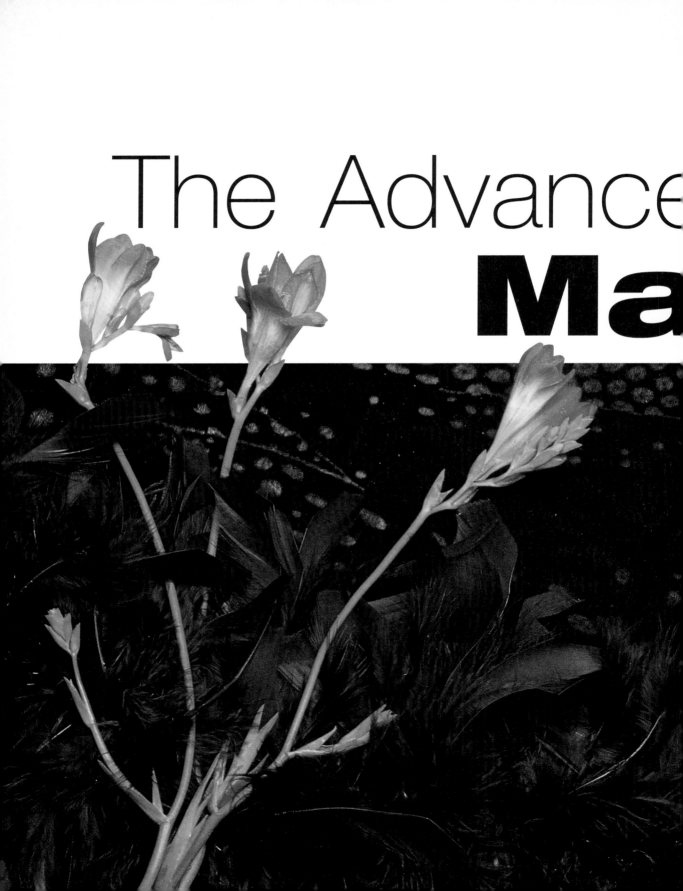

The Advance
Ma

keover

Are you open to the myriad measures available today to transform yourself radically? Before we look at the ways in which you can sort out the bits that bug you, let's be sure you are ready for a radical revamp.

No treatment, therapy or makeover changes the real person – that's you, inside. If you think that by having breast implants or liposuction on your thighs your life will change and you will attract the man of your dreams, forget it. Any problem or unhappiness needs to be dealt with separately and appropriately, with you recognizing the root causes and finding a way to put it right. By looking different, even lots better, you might feel more confident but the problems will still be there.

In this chapter we will explore ways to change yourself radically. A few options cost nothing – like changing your voice. Others are also free but require real effort – like getting your body into better shape. Some, however, demand a healthy bank balance – such as cosmetic or dental surgery. You might shudder at the idea of having surgery for cosmetic rather than health reasons, but for many women (and men) such alternatives have helped.

Delve into all the possibilities for an advanced makeover with an open mind. If you aren't ready for any of it today, you might be one day soon.

Radical style surgery

Does your wardrobe reflect the woman that you are today and the woman that you want to be? Perhaps your job requires a 'uniformed' look Monday to Friday that doesn't express the real you. Does looking like someone else affect your self-esteem and morale? If so, should you be pursuing other options for a new work environment that might allow you to be you?

Many women can get thrown into turmoil when their circumstances change – a new job, a new home, losing/gaining a partner, having/losing children. When your life changes, for better or worse, it's good to take a look in the mirror, after the dust has settled, and ask yourself if it's time now that you changed as well.

Divorce or losing a partner creates the ultimate upheaval. Becoming single again, after many years in a couple, is odd. You know you have now to make it on your own and you may realize that your attitude and your image need a revamp so that you face the world afresh as an individual.

New Attitude,
New Self

SUE There are women who talk about getting fit and there are others who actually do it. Sue is one of the latter.

Watching the London Marathon on television one year, Sue said, 'I'm going to do that one day.' Her family fell about in fits of laughter: Sue was then fifteen stone and led a sedentary life during which she sometimes ate without even being aware of it, one or two cream cakes with coffee each day perhaps, and a few pints of beer in the evening in addition to regular meals. 'Before I knew it, I was buying dresses in size 24.'

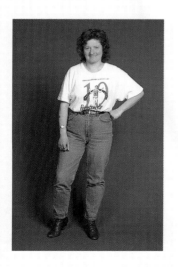

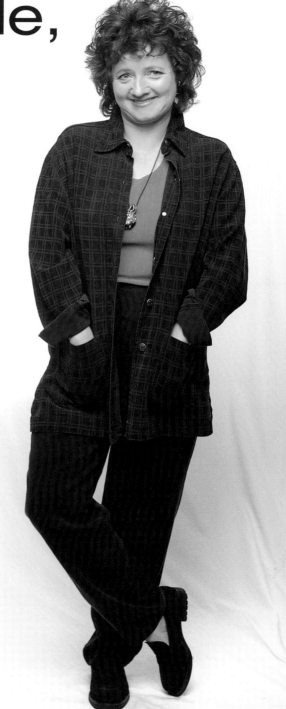

With her husband, Sue joined the local gym and was surprised to enjoy the treadmill. From there, Sue progressed to running around the block, joined by her son running backwards alongside her and laughing!

Determined she could sustain the running, Sue changed her whole lifestyle to accelerate weight loss. She cut out all the junk in her diet along with the alcohol and was amazed by how the pounds fell away without her ever weighing food portions or counting calories. In addition, Sue abandoned her car and started cycling sixteen miles back and forth to work each day.

Sue shed a total of five stone in less than a year and began shopping in 'real' shops again, not ones exclusively for the fuller figure. With the change in body shape and fitness came a new self-confidence, but her marriage was put under strain. Her husband did not like the new positive Sue, who was making friends and developing interests. Sue stayed motivated and kept training, and eventually she and her husband split. Before long, among her new friends was a special man who helped her through her first marathon. Sue has now completed the London Marathon not once, but three times.

THE RESULT Like many formerly overweight women, Sue's been at a loss to know how to make the most of her new figure. Once she threw away all her tent dresses she went straight to jeans and T-shirts. But Sue's curvy, hourglass shape isn't flattered in stiff, constricting jeans, and as her wardrobe is mainly black she wanted ideas for good colour. Her bright Celtic colouring sparkles in clear fun colours. In the right colour, we notice Sue first and her clothes afterwards. Soft, drapy fabrics not only complement a curvy figure but are slimming as well.

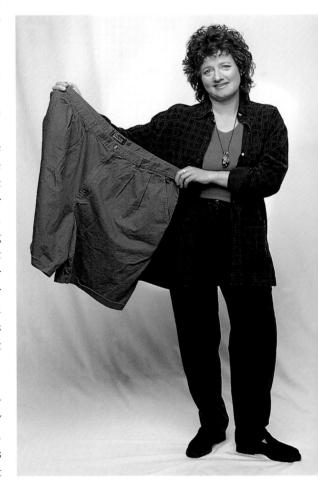

Change Your Body:
Cosmetic Surgery

If you are so bothered by a less than perfect feature, you might consider one of the many surgical techniques available to remove or reshape your personal bugbear. Hey, if Roseanne Barr, Elizabeth Taylor, Tom Cruise and countless other people in the public eye can do it with such success, why not you?

If you want to forgo a holiday this (and, possibly, next) year, or if you receive an unexpected windfall from an aunt or in this year's bonus, why not consider one of the new approaches to eliminating that one frustration you face every day in the mirror? Women and men have gained tremendous confidence from straightening that crooked nose or pinning down those protruding ears.

Is surgery right for you?

Cosmetic surgery is not for everyone. It has risks. You must shop around not only for a qualified surgeon (this is not as straightforward as it should be) but also for one who gives you confidence.

First stop must be a consultation with your own doctor. If you have heard about a surgeon from a friend or in an article, have your GP check out his qualifications. When choosing a plastic surgeon, enquire about his/her skills in cosmetic surgery. Someone who spends time repairing unfortunate accident victims might not be the most skilled or up to date with cosmetic surgery.

In meeting with a surgeon, watch for signs of pressure from him/her. Any clinic that applies pressure, however subtle, to get you to commit to a procedure before you are ready is not to be trusted. Find out all the possible side effects so that you know what to expect in the hours, days and weeks after surgery.

Meet with two or three surgeons to be sure you are selecting the best one for you. Although you will be charged for each consultation, you will learn a great deal at each one and be better informed as a result.

There are many different procedures on offer. The most popular ones are described here.

Facial options

A nose job: Otherwise known as rhinoplasty, nose jobs are done under a general anaesthetic. As the surgery is internal there is no scarring. The procedure can help to improve your breathing (or reduce your snoring!) if your problems result from an excess of cartilage inside the nose. Modest reshaping to repair a break or a major transformation to give you the nose of your dreams are both possible. Be prepared for discomfort for five to seven days while you endure a splint inside your nose.

A chin job: For mentoplasty, or a chin job, a silicone implant is inserted through a fine line under the chin. The effect can be subtle but make a profound difference to a receding chin. Minimal discomfort, and recovery takes about a week. A similar procedure is also available for the cheeks.

An eye job: Blepharoplasty can be performed on the upper lid to eliminate excess skin that causes droopy eyes, or on the lower lid/under-eye area to get rid of bags (of fat, usually) and wrinkles. Expect to look like you've gone a few rounds with Frank Bruno for up to two weeks and to appreciate the full results in about six to eight weeks.

Ear correction: Octoplasty is a procedure to pin down protruding ears and can be done at any age. Very quick recovery of only five to seven days.

Endoscopic facial surgery: This is keyhole surgery for the face. An endoscope (surgical telescope) is inserted into small holes around the hairline and inside the mouth, allowing the surgeon to reposition the tissue in the face and brow. You can opt for a brow lift or a face lift with this method, but it is effective only if the sagging is minimal and so is better on younger faces. Recovery from the brow lift takes about seven to ten days; for the face lift, about two weeks. There may be some damage to the nerves in the forehead and scalp, causing some permanent numbness.

Full face or mask lift: Here incisions are made inside the mouth and around the face from ear to ear, with the surgeon stretching and repositioning facial tissue. This produces the 'wow' before-and-after pictures and is for women who won't benefit from the more minor endoscopic procedure. As this is a major operation, expect to take up to eight weeks to see the full benefit.

Skin-peeling and laser treatments: These are for women keen to transform surface wrinkles and fine lines, discoloration (such as age spots) or scarred skin (such as from acne). Check the credentials of any clinic offering this service as you need to ensure that the medical back-up is as sound as with surgery.

Skin peeling uses high concentrations of glycolic or lactic acids or Retin-A. The practitioner must test your tolerance to any chemical peeling agent before proceeding with a full peel.

Dermabrasion brushes off the top layers of skin and is especially effective on scarred or sun-damaged skin. Be prepared to go into hiding for a month or more as the raw surface is eventually replaced with fresh, clear new skin. Total sunblock is essential for the first six months as you will be highly susceptible to burning and further damage if exposed to the sun.

Laser treatments (or resurfacing) shine laser light over the surface of the skin to burn away the top layers. This can be done in spots such as under the eye or around the mouth. But as new skin is of a very different texture to old skin and these regions will look red and sore for three to four weeks, consider the benefits of doing the whole face at once.

Body options

The Breasts

Breast reduction: A godsend to women weary of carrying heavy breasts. The operation removes excess breast tissue via an incision either under the breast or around the nipple (which is replaced at the end). Best to consider after childbearing.

Breast lifting: The answer for the bra-burning babes who regret not wearing the proper support for so long and who now have droopy, pendulous breasts without any tone. Also only worth considering after having children.

Breast augmentation: Favoured by the many famous 'have-nots'. Silicone, saline or soya implants are inserted under the breast tissue, leaving a nominal scar. The latest triluscent (soya) implants, which can be scanned by a mammogram, are considered to be state of the art and are preferable to the troublesome silicone implants, which are still subject to legal claims and have been linked to a weakening of the immune system.

Fat Removal

Liposuction and liposculpture: Although there are women who resort to the surgical removal of fat rather than persevere with exercise or sensible eating, this procedure is really meant for stubborn areas of fat that you've either inherited or just can't shift. Any part of the body where fat forms can be treated, from the face and neck to the breasts, tummy, thigh and bottom, even to the ankles.

Liposuction should be pursued only as a last resort and by a highly qualified and experienced doctor. The catalogue of horrors from procedures gone wrong are regularly reported in the women's magazines. But it can be beneficial for some. Recovery takes about a week, with swelling and bruising lasting up to four weeks, after which time you will see the benefits.

Non-surgical wonders

Facial exercises: I first met and worked with Eva Fraser years ago, and I have seen the effects of her disciplined routine on both her and myself. Her exercises are easy to follow and can be incorporated into a regular routine or practised during 'dead' times, such as when watching TV or stuck in a traffic jam.

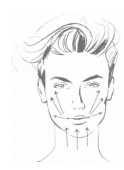

The Neck, Jaw & Face Lift

A saggy neck and jaw not only make us appear older but also severe or even unfriendly. This exercise will work to firm under the chin and neck and lift the muscles in the lower face and cheeks.

♦ Sit straight with square shoulders. Now jut the jaw forward so that the neck is stretched.
♦ Open the mouth by just dropping the jaw. Extend jaw slowly out lifting the bottom teeth over the upper teeth.
♦ Lift bottom lip as if to touch your nose.
♦ In this position smile upwards slowly in 5 definite steps in the directions marked. Hold for 5 counts. Lower in 5 definite steps.
♦ Repeat 3 times daily.

The Winning Smile (1)

To fight the jolly jowls of ageing here are two simple exercises to ensure your smile remains beautiful.

♦ Mouth closed with teeth together but relaxed. No other facial muscles must be tense; particularly around the eyes.
♦ With the lips and teeth together smile widely in the direction of the arrows in 5 definite steps.
♦ At the broadest point hold for 10 counts. Return the smile in 5 definite steps.
♦ Repeat 3 times daily.

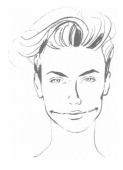

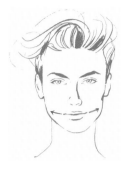

The Winning Smile (2)

With age we can start to appear 'down in the mouth'. But these muscles can be easily exercised to lift the corners giving you a more cheerful, younger and smoother appearance.

♦ Teeth together and lips closed. No facial tension anywhere.
♦ Work one side of the mouth at a time. Smile to one side, lifting the corner of the mouth in 5 definite steps in the direction of the arrow.
♦ Hold for 5 counts whilst you try to push your cheek muscles up to almost close the eye. Return in 5 definite steps. Repeat for the opposite side.
♦ Repeat this exercise 3 times on each side daily.

The Eye Opener

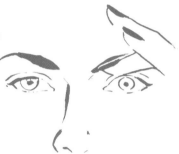

Age and gravity take a toll on the eyes. The lids and underbrow area can start to droop even before you reach 30! This 'Eye Opener' exercise is a sure cure for the droops when practised regularly and done properly.

♦ Rest elbows on a firm surface. Working on both eyes together curve the index finger slightly and place along the orbital bone.
♦ With a firm press, lift the muscles and pull up and out.
♦ Look straight ahead and close the lids slowly. Squeeze lids shut to 6 counts.
♦ Once closed, tightly squeeze eyelids for 3 counts.
♦ Open lids and relax. Repeat 3 times daily.

Micro-current massage: This uses electrical probes to boost the blood circulation while firming the muscles. The more toned the facial muscles, the smoother the skin appears, with wrinkles less apparent. A one-hour session can give the face a glow, but up to six sessions are required for the treatment to be effective.

Electrical injection: A sterile needle is targeted at fine lines to stimulate the production of collagen and elastin. Rollers are then used to plump out the skin. The procedure takes up to two hours and is effective on specific areas such as the upper lip and brow.

CACI: The original non-surgical face lift, this uses a low-frequency microcurrent to strengthen and tighten the support muscles of the face and to improve the general condition of the skin and connective tissues. A great way to zap yourself into better condition, but it requires a dozen or so sessions to see real (albeit short-term) results.

Salon therapies: Many salons offer 'the latest and greatest' approaches to massaging the skin with the supposed results of better tone and texture. Such attentive pampering, with beautifully smelling plant extracts, undoubtedly makes you feel better and look radiant.

Investing in a Smile

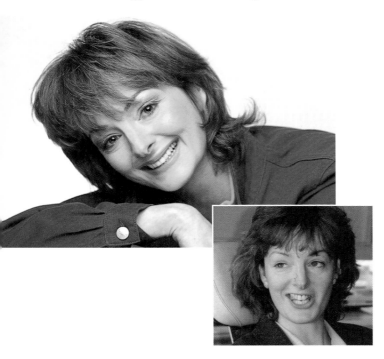

JULIA Whenever I suggest that someone postpone their holidays and have dental work instead, I am usually greeted with a millisecond of shock followed by enthusiastic concurrence. Often I am told, 'I wish someone had suggested that years ago.'

Julia finally took the plunge and consulted one of London's top dental surgeons after one of her sons commented on holiday about the state of her teeth.

'Mummy,' he said, 'you look better if you don't smile. Your teeth are horrible.' Julia explained: 'I have had a variety of work done on my teeth since I was young. Along with some badly receding gums and darkening teeth in front, I now have a mouth full of amalgam fillings. The fillings have to be replaced eventually so I have opted to get the whole lot sorted properly – for my boys as well as myself.'

Dentist Neil Lawson-Baker confirms that the condition of your teeth affects your personality. 'I have seen both women and men go on to become much more effective communicators just because they finally got the confidence to use their mouths fully. Julia's situation is not uncommon. Many women in their thirties who have had inadequate dental care earlier in life need to take remedial steps to keep decay in check and to replace discoloured caps, implants or fillings.'

Now that Julia has invested in cosmetic dentistry, her smile is a pleasure for everyone, especially her sons, to behold. And all she needs now is an update to her look, to warrant flashing that smile as often as possible.

As a busy mother and executive wife,

Throat: The quality of your sounds is affected by how well you use your throat. Many of us restrict the use of the throat (and the mouth), effectively strangling the words and sounds. Singing is a great release for a constricted throat. You know you sound heaps more like Celine Dion if you widen the back of your throat and let those notes sail out. To speak well, you don't need to go to such extremes, but try to open up the throat so that the sounds reverberate to come over as rich as possible. An open throat requires a relaxed jaw and flexible facial muscles, which helps to ease the mouth and throat. The throat then 'feels' capable of more expansive, fuller sound.

Mouth and face: A stiff upper lip cannot produce a rich voice or make words sound magical. Many adults have indifferent voices because their mouths and faces are stiff and hardly move. If you have good breathing, diction and articulation but you use your mouth as a funnel, you won't have a compelling voice. Try to open up your face, mouth and jaw when you speak. Do so, in a very exaggerated fashion, in front of a mirror. Have a laugh. Work your face, mouth and jaw like an animated speaker you admire. Dawn French, Sharon Stone, Joanna Lumley, Andie McDowell, Gloria Hunniford, Ruby Wax, Goldie Hawn and Bette Midler all make full use of their face, mouth and jaw and have rich, distinctive voices as a result.

The sound of your
own voice

If you want to improve your voice, you need to start by analysing it. Take a tape recorder and read something from the newspaper or talk about your day into it. Play the tape back. Note what you like and what you don't. Keep the original recording to see how your voice improves as you continue to practise speaking better, using better diction, varying the pitch and pace, and improving the general quality.

Imitate characteristics in others that you like. For example, a colleague at work might sound quite impressive to you because she speaks more loudly than you do. Imitate her and turn up your volume. Watching a movie, you might note how another voice has variety and isn't monotone (as yours might be). Try 'acting' the new voice with your tape recorder by reading a story for a few minutes, trying to imitate the pitch of the voice you admire. If you hear a change – and you like it – keep practising. Start to use your new techniques every time you speak and soon they will be your voice.

Changing your accent

Practising can result in change. I grew up in a part of America (Boston, Massachusetts) that has a broad, distinctive accent. At the age of ten I moved to the New York region, where people spoke differently. I felt like a hick. I come from a large family, the Bostonian accent thrived at home, and my mother was adamant that we retained our regional accents. But I hated the sound of it and suffered playground taunting because of it.

At fourteen, I mustered the courage to ask my English teacher for help and over a few months she worked with me to wipe out the broadest bits of my accent while sparing me the worst twangs of

New York. Accents add colour and personality to speech. But when an accent prevents you from being intelligible and communicating effectively with the people around you, work is required to edit out the quirkiest bits.

I have worked with politicians and business people on their voices as part of presentation training, I have urged several to work on two levels to make their accents more effective. First, restrict the use of colloquialisms that won't be understood by others. Secondly, be more conscious of your diction, and take care to enunciate carefully. If you do these two things, while keeping your regional accent, you will be accepted by all and be an effective communicator.

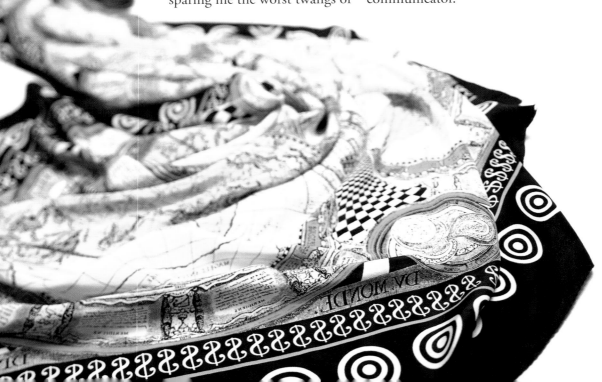

A New Partner:
How to Attract the Man of Your Dreams

A motivation often cited for doing something really radical about one's image stems from being dissatisfied with one's love life. If you too are convinced that if only you looked, sounded or behaved differently you would meet men more easily, then maybe it is time you considered the ways to revamp your thinking about making yourself attractive to the man of your dreams.

Finding Mr Wonderful might be easier than you think. Nothing saddens me more than a woman desperate for companionship and love who writes herself off as never being able to find a good man. Supermen appear out of the blue only in the movies. In real life, although surprises do happen, you have to make your own happiness, or else grow old waiting hopefully for him to materialize.

If you want to find a new partner, first you have to define him, and then find him. In developing his profile, keep asking yourself if you are the kind of woman to attract him. If not, what steps are required to recreate yourself, to expand the possibilities for your own personality and image and to lure Mr Wonderful?

Dating agencies and personal columns are the obvious vehicles to which lonely hearts often resort. While many have found happiness via both, it takes a lot of courage, panache and perseverance, not to mention money, to go through the sifting process until you find a soulmate. If you don't fit the most marketable profile – under 35 and childless – why not be more creative in finding some potential male friends, if not future lovers?

Defining him

He's there in your dreams: make him realilty. So get two pieces of paper and set out the following headings on each: Personality, Career, Interests, Passions and Looks. One page is for him, the other is for you.

Personality

Do you want an outgoing man or someone more introspective? Is he to be a touchy-feelie type who likes to talk things through and share his innermost thoughts, or do you prefer a more stiff-upper-lip type, who needs coaxing to reveal his true self? Is your ideal companion a natural comedian or someone who will appreciate your inclination to perform? Just write down at random the various characteristics you seek.

Now see how much your personality mirrors these traits. Consider how you might need to adapt your own personality to attract someone like him. If you want that personality type in a man badly enough, you can work to become more like him yourself or to become the kind of woman who would complement him.

Career

Mr Wonderful's career may matter a great deal to you. It's too easy to stereotype different careers, so be careful you don't make unwise judgements and write off, say, an accountant because you think he'll be a bore. I've met some pretty wild accountants!

Doctors, plumbers and artists don't necessarily hang out together or congregate at predictable places. But, if the career is important, be clever at finding ways to meet his type. Don't worry if your work is the opposite of his or supposedly below or above his in status. Just be prepared to show an interest in his work once you meet. As all women know, men define themselves by their work and, initially, love to talk about little else.

Finding your man by his career requires a bit of ingenuity. Say, for instance, you seek an entrepreneur. Follow the business pages in the local newspaper to find out about successful new start-up ventures in the area. Once identified, why not approach a few 'candidates' to discuss their contributing to a local community charity or project to enhance their profile? When you meet the man, you can determine his availability and his desirability. One meeting could lead to another. Casually suggest you meet somewhere socially to discuss details of the project further. You would simply be employing basic business practices, which he will find familiar, but have the dual objective of mixing a good cause with your business.

Regardless of your credentials, you can always find a way to meet a man within a certain field if you put your mind to it. Try visiting local, regional or national exhibitions that might attract his type. For example, travel and computer exhibitions attract a broad range of different men. Once there, use your charm to ask clever questions of a few desirable targets. What's more natural than meeting someone new and discussing a common interest? Just make sure you aren't totally out of your depth before you open your mouth.

As all men love to feel like experts, start by asking if he could direct you to someone who could explain something, and soon, expert or not, he'll be doing his best to show off all he knows. I use this trick at gardening shows – just for the fun of it, mind you (my husband might get the wrong idea) – and I find it doesn't take too long before an offer of coffee comes up.

Interests

These are easy to define and should either be your own or ones that you would like to develop. If you're keen to travel but have yet to spread your wings, go for it. There are many holidays geared around an activity such as walking, golfing, tennis or painting, even for the absolute beginner. Go on your own and you will be sure to meet several men who share the same interests.

Passions

Unlike interests, passions cannot be contrived. What makes you tremble with excitement (like jazz or opera, modern art, antiques, gardening, food, and so on) or so angry you could scream (such as a social cause, endangered wildlife/animals or a particular illness)? Follow your passion, join appropriate societies, get involved

and you will meet men who share your intensity of feeling for the same cause. What better way to light a spark between two people?

Looks

These are the final consideration, and not to be dismissed if we are truly honest. If your Mr Wonderful is youthful and vibrant, so too must you be to attract him. If you aren't, consider the measures necessary to become someone he would notice.

How does he dress? If he's to be elegant, possibly conservative, will your bohemian style scare him off? If, like so many men, he's a bit unconscious about his style, how can you attract him without seeming to be 'off limits'. You'd be surprised how many men are terrified of making the first move towards an attractive woman.

Finding Mr Wonderful might seem like a lot of work. But even if you don't find the man you've described, you are bound to find another who makes your dream Mr Wonderful pale by comparison. Just think of what fun you'll have in the pursuit. Happy hunting!

The Colour
Ma

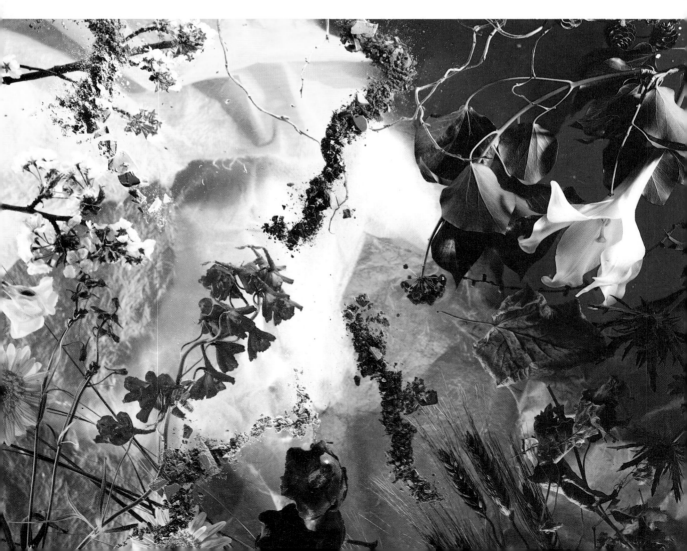

keover

If you want to make a big difference to your look, try colour analysis. Wearing your best colours will dramatically affect your appearance. People won't be able to say what is different about you, just that you look terrific. You can look better, even healthier, in the right coloured clothes without wearing any or much make-up.

Color Me Beautiful started a revolution in 1980 when it launched its colour theory on the world. The premise was, and remains, that if you wear colours that complement your skin tone, eye and hair colouring, you look more natural and healthy. Since then, we have colour-analysed millions of people around the world and have continued to fine-tune and improve our approach over the years.

When a woman has a colour analysis, she is excited about the prospect of looking better than she ever imagined. We develop colour prejudices when we are young, reinforced by what Mum or our friends liked, then dictated by fashion, and we invariably end up with a wardrobe of a few tried and tested winners alongside a multitude of losers.

Colour analysis simplifies all that by showing you a range of colours (which represent hundreds more) and giving you a set of fabric swatches to guide you when shopping. I know, I know. Many colour-analysed women, despite our advice not to, follow those colours a bit too religiously and refuse to buy anything unless it matches their swatches exactly. Our goal is to make shopping easier, not more difficult.

Our principles still hold true but we approach colour analysis differently today than we did back then. We realize that even though a range of colours may 'technically' be right for a woman, they just might not be her. She must be fully involved for us to find her best palette. A colour analysis that dictates without discussion is faulty.

For example, many fair, blue-eyed blondes look gorgeous in one of our Light palettes but want more drama than those colours necessarily provide. We have to accept that they will still want to wear black or navy, and must show them how to do so to best effect.

We also know that women want to look current, part of today. Every fashion season thrills and annoys us at the same time with the array of shades on offer. The colour-aware shopper knows how to compromise intelligently with colour, that is, to make fashionable colours work with her palette because the style of the clothes is just what she needs and wants.

So if you are 'colour blind', either through sticking too rigidly to your range of colours or through never having discovered the full possibilities available to you, it's time to wise up.

'Like mother, like daughter'

Often a woman's attitude towards colour is shaped by her mother. 'I can't wear that colour. My mother always said I looked dreadful in it.' Or, if mum said it was a killer when you were young, you now have a wardrobe full of it just out of spite.

Indeed this syndrome extends beyond families to friends, because we are all prejudiced by the colours we like and often fail to appreciate how special or different they

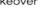

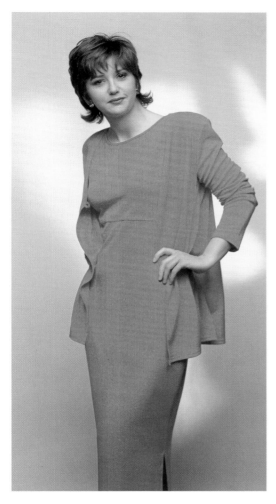

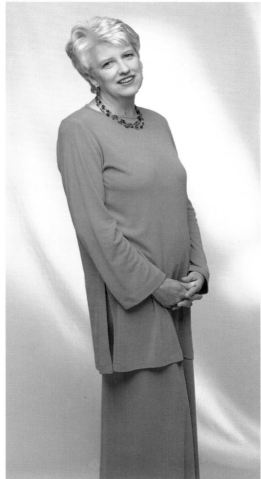

can be on others. That's why it is often fatal to shop with a sister or friend, for they might get all excited about a great colour and you get caught up in their excitement only to end up looking unsuccessful in it whilst your mate looks a million.

Kate and Julie are a beautiful mother and daughter team. Both have similar body shapes, although Kate's, at mid-life, is understandably a size or two bigger than young Julie's. But whilst they can both wear the same styles, they should never share clothes because their colouring is quite opposite. Julie has inherited her dad's warmer colouring, while Kate looks winning in cooler tones.

Fine-Tuning Your
Colours

Many women found that knowing their best colours was both liberating and, in a sense, restrictive. They are freed from fashion pressures about the 'latest colours' and only select what they know is a winner on them personally, but sometimes they are so devoted to their palettes that they adhere to them too rigidly, without knowing ways in which to wear them to look more current.

SARAH Sarah has loved her wonderful rich, warm, Deep Autumn colours and never bored of them. But going grey has thrown her into turmoil. The first white hairs appeared in her twenties and now, at thirty-three, she has a thick strip of white around her face, which she covers regularly with a semi-permanent rinse.

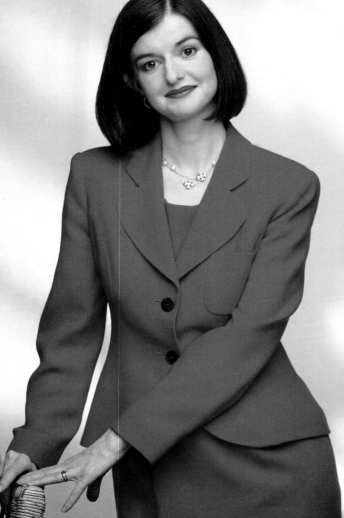

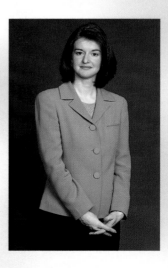

'My image consultant recommended that I soften my colours now that I am greying,' she explained. As you get older, softer versions of favourite colours are often more flattering. But premature grey does not mean that your overall looks are ageing. Both camel and red are terrific on Sarah, but she still looks better in strong colours. She wears black, red, olive or navy to best effect.

I think women like Sarah should keep the grey at bay until it is too much of a hassle to keep covering – at that point, go for the glorious salt and pepper look. We sought the advice of colour specialists Wella. They suggested that Sarah weave a permanent tint over the grey area and gloss up the rest of her hair with a semi-permanent rinse. The permanent tint would need redoing after two months, and the semi-permanent after one month. The semi-permanent would keep any sprouting grey hairs or any grey roots at bay.

EMILY 'Having my colours done a few years ago changed my life,' says Emily, a forty-something mother, wife and country-woman. She used to wear camels and browns with a mixture of pinks and navies. Colour coordination was a big problem. 'I just couldn't believe how simple it was to get a scheme to help you look great and to get everything to work together so easily.'

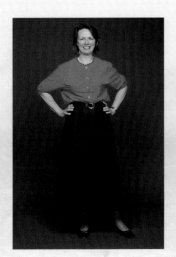

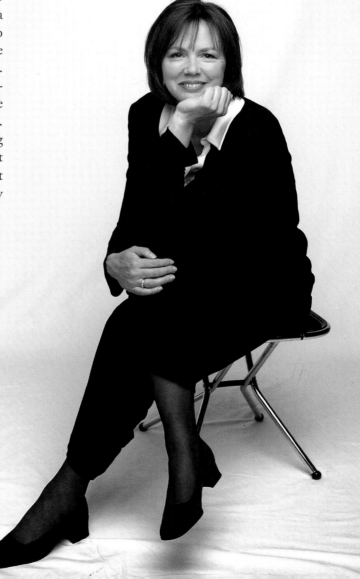

Learning that she suited rich, soft, 'cooler' colours meant Emily could develop a colour scheme in those tones. Out went all the browns, moss greens and beiges.

Emily wanted clothes ideas for evening suppers with friends, when she likes to put away the practical gear and look feminine. 'But I am really very classic and don't like fussy clothes,' she explained.

Knitted, washable separates are the answer to looking smart while still being able to do the dishes – and Emily loved these (so much so that she went out and bought the outfit!). Shoulder pads may come and go in fashion, but for women like Emily with sloping shoulders they can make all the difference between looking 'good' and looking 'fantastic'.

Then it was time to update her colours. We told Emily to toss out the hot pink lipstick for a while (it was looking pretty dated) and use softer matte raspberry tones, which look more current. Navy is Emily's best neutral. When you find a great style in a great neutral for you, don't hesitate to buy it.

Colour basics

There are, no doubt, basic colours already in your wardrobe that form its foundation. Neutral colours – black, charcoal, navy, brown, stone, taupe, camel and beige – are readily found in the widest range of garments, fabrics and styles. But a few of these may be very unflattering if worn too close to the face on the wrong woman.

Black: Drains all but the most striking or well made-up women.

Beige: Makes many women look in need of a pint of blood if not helped along with another hue.

Camel: Looks rich on a woman with warm skin tone and hair but looks inexpensive on someone with cool, rosy colouring.

Brown: Comes in a host of shades from almost black through to terracotta, cinnamon, coffee and cocoa. The savvy woman knows that only one or two versions of brown are her best and doesn't buy a mixture.

White: The final, key basic is your version of white. You should have discovered by now which white is best on you, that is, can be worn alone near your face. Pure crisp white is best on dark skins but also suits the 'Snow Whites' with porcelain skin and dark hair. Other women look much healthier in a Soft White, Ivory or Oyster. The fabric you choose for your whites also plays a part in helping it work or fail. Linen, knits and jersey, because they are matte, are softer on the face than the sheen of silk, satin or polyester.

The following pages present wardrobe schemes for the different colouring types. Each of these can be taken in new directions – cooler or warmer, brighter or softer, lighter or deeper – depending on your hair colour (if you change it) and your personality. If a palette seems a bit subdued but does describe you best, consider how you could add some punch without straying too far. The beauty of working with one palette is that the colours co-ordinate beautifully, thus making your clothing investments greater value and you wardrobe more manageable.

The Right Choice

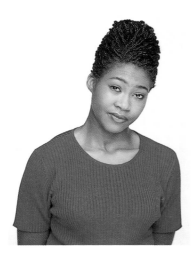

JANICE Women with strong natural colouring must do themselves justice with the colours they choose. Black skins 'absorb' make-up colours designed for Caucasians and benefit from using lines designed for their own beauty needs. So, too, they need to be sure that the colours for their clothes make them look marvellous.

Janice is so pretty that she looks good in lots of colours. But why look good when you can look great? Powdery colours like this dusty blue are not strong enough to make her sparkle. But a bright, true blue does the job beautifully.

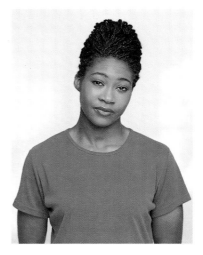

The Light Wardrobe

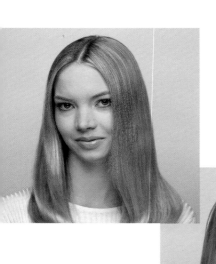

Successful

In soft, delicate pastels you look fresh and bright. But take care that light colours in shiny fabrics aren't too electric against your face.

Least successful

Your blonde hair might contrast well with a dark colour like navy but the overall effect on your face is not flattering. In black or navy you can look very tired, even unwell.

Overall impression

Fair/pale

Color Me Beautiful season

Light Spring or Light Summer

Famous examples

Zoë Ball; Goldie Hawn; Claudia Schiffer

Goals

Not to overwhelm your colouring with very strong or deep colours and high-contrast patterns. When wearing black, expose skin at the neckline or soften with another colour

Helpful hints

If you look pale in a colour it is probably too dark or too bright for you

Make-up advice

Eyes

Navy, teal, grey or taupe shadows; apricot, soft pink or melon highlighter

Brows

Cocoa or taupe brown

Liner

Navy, grey, teal; soften with taupe or cocoa shadow

Mascara

Brown or navy

Blush

Pale pink, peach, salmon

Lipstick

Most pale pinks (warm or cool); clear red

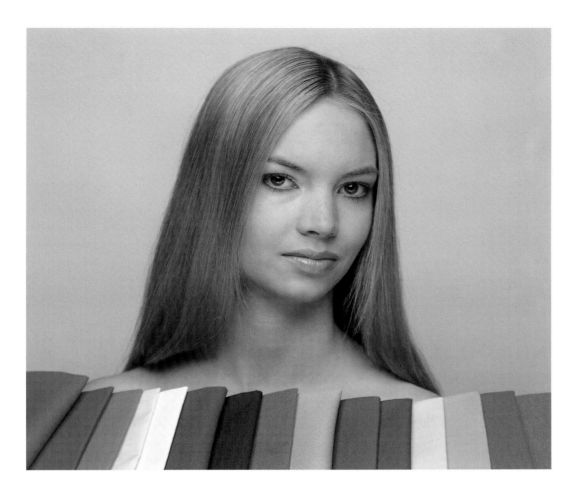

Colours to wear

Here is a selection of shades for building a great wardrobe to suit you. The basics include soft white, pale or medium blues, aquas and teals, pinks, violets, pearl greys and fresh reds like watermelon. That navy is actually a soft, light version and best on you with a pastel or red rather than white.

Add to these colours extra warmer tones if they flatter you, such as camel, peach shades and warm pinks, along with soft moss greens. Butter-milk, ivory and light yellows will also be terrific.

If you know that cooler tones (blue-based colours) compliment you, add pewter, rose brown, mints and pastel blue-greens, along with lilacs and burgundy.

The Deep Wardrobe

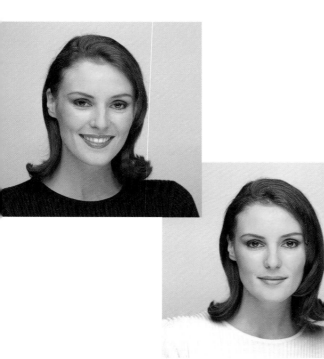

Successful

Think Snow White and you've got the look. Deep rich colours such as black, navy or chocolate brown are dramatic winners. Always choose the deepest, truest versions to look your best.

Least successful

Soft pastels aren't bad on you but they aren't terrific. If you have plenty in your wardrobe, team them with striking jackets or scarves, or just start to replace colours like these, which are insipid on you, with better ones.

Overall impression

Strong and rich

Color Me Beautiful season

Deep Autumn or Deep Winter

Famous examples

Paloma Picasso; Naomi Campbell; Teri Hatcher

Goals

To complement your rich looks with vibrant shades, bold contrasts or striking solid blocks of colour

Helpful hints

Make indifferent, neutral shades look more interesting by wearing a deep contrast (black, deep brown, navy)

Make-up advice

Eyes

Navy, spruce, plum, charcoal; ivory, apricot or icy pink as highlighter

Brows

Grey/brown to blend with natural colour

Liner

Black, navy, pine, plum; keep intensity by covering with a matching or deep shadow

Mascara

Black, plum, navy

Blush

Terracotta or salmon to warm up your look; plum to work with cooler pink lipsticks; soft 'red' blush when wearing red lipstick

Lipstick

Mahogany and terracotta for warm look; plum, raspberry, hot pink for cool look; true red

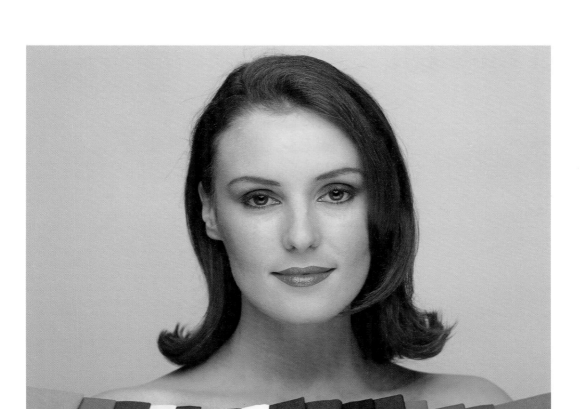

Colours to wear

With strong colouring you need to go for rich, true colours. Your wardrobe should have clean, crisp white; primary versions of red, blue, green and yellow; mahogany, pine, mango, teal, turquoise and purple. You probably don't need telling that you are a stunner in black as well as inky navy, charcoal, deepest brown and pewter.

You can push your wardrobe palette warmer by adding terracotta, rust, olive, bronze and other golden deep tones if you know that they flatter you.

Or, to move into a cooler direction, add blue reds, hot pinks and icy pastels. Think white with just a dash of colour.

The Cool Wardrobe

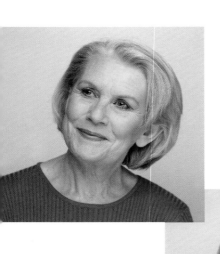

Successful

You do not need to spend a fortune to look terrific and younger. Just choose the right colour. Pink- or blue-based plum is a winner if your colouring is cool.

Least successful

Beware of warm colours, even if they are fashionable, when your colouring is so cool. You will only look tired and older. Who needs that?

Overall impression

Rosy/grey

Color Me Beautiful season

Cool Summer, Cool Winter

Famous examples

Betty Boothroyd, Joan Baez, Queen Elizabeth II

Goals

To complement your pinky, soft complexion and cool grey hair

Helpful hints

Avoid yellow, green and brown undertones. Only pinky browns like cocoa will be good, unlike beige, khaki or golden brown

Make-up advice

Eyes

Soft navy, smoky grey, plum, pine; ivory or pale pink as highlighter

Brows

Cocoa or taupe

Liner

Navy, pine, plum; softened with a stroke of grey or taupe eye shadow over the top

Mascara

Navy or black

Blush

Rose, plum, soft burgundy

Lipstick

Raspberry, dusty rose, hot pink, soft fuchsia

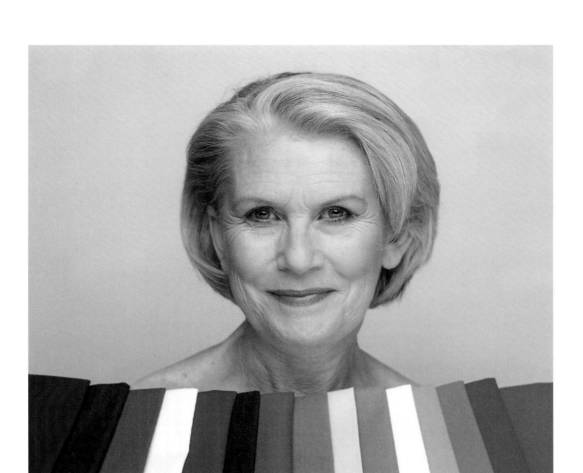

Colours to wear

Your possibilities for looking terrific are many. No browns in sight aside from cocoa or a rose brown. Most shades of blue are fine, but stop short of overpowering royals, which are too strong.

All greys are winners, and your best choice for neutral basics over anything warm like camel. Violets can be the lightest lilacs (great with navy, charcoal or soft white) or the richest periwinkle.

Reds are wonderful, especially if blue-based or clear. Try red instead of black for the evening.

The Warm Wardrobe

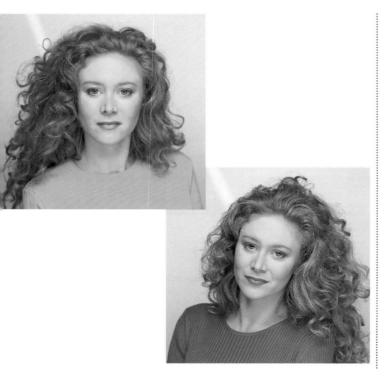

Successful

With such striking golden colouring, you need to be sure that the undertones of all your clothes complement you. When it comes to pink, think salmon, coral, peach or mango.

Least successful

You might see redheads in cool colours in fashion magazines, but in real life redheads look harsh and artificial dressed 'coolly', even when young and beautiful. What hope is there for real golden gals when they try to wear shades that are ghastly on them?

Overall impression

Golden (rich or fair)

Color Me Beautiful seasons

Warm Spring, Warm Autumn

Famous Examples

Sarah, Duchess of York; Nicole Kidman; Lulu

Goals

To complement your warm skin tone and hair colour with rich, warm tones

Helpful hints

Avoid pure white in favour of ivory. Try to 'warm up' stark outfits like black or navy with a better colour near your face, such as terracotta, golden yellow or salmon

Make-up advice

Eyes

Brown, olive, moss or teal; apricot or melon for highlighter

Brows

Warm brown to blend with your own brows

Liner

Teal, olive, purple; for a softer look brush over with a soft brown shadow

Mascara

Brown

Blush

Apricot, salmon or terracotta

Lipstick

Orange red, warm pinks, terracotta

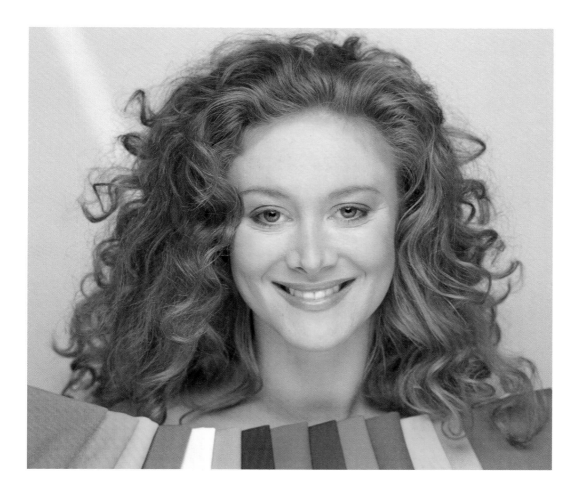

Colours to wear

A warm wardrobe should be filled with more than just browns and beiges. Your whites are ivory or cream: pure white is an absolute killer against your skin tone and hair.

Your greens are moss, bronze and olive. Blues can look cheap on you (unless you have blue eyes). Better bets will be the aquas, turquoise tones and teal blues.

Keep your yellows creamy or golden and wear them with anything you consider too harsh on its own, such as black or navy. Avoid greys in favour of camel, golden brown and rust as good investment neutrals. Don't forget tomato red, even if your hair is red!

The Soft Wardrobe

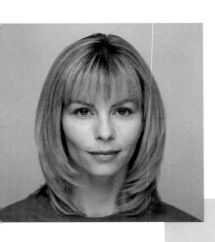

Successful

Muted colours are anything but dull on women with soft colouring. Whether light or deep, as long as they are 'greyed down' they will be winners.

Least successful

You might like the colour but does it like you back? Here's a perfect example of a colour wearing you, not the reverse.

Overall impression

Muted/mousy

Color Me Beautiful seasons

Soft Summer, Soft Autumn

Famous examples

Jennifer Aniston, Cindy Crawford, Hillary Clinton

Goals

Not to overpower your look in very bright colours or stark contrasts

Helpful hints

Blended colours, monochromatic shades and matte fabrics are your best options

Make-up advice

Eyes

Charcoal, deep brown, soft plum, spruce; melon or apricot as highlighter

Brows

Taupe to blend with your own colour

Liner

Charcoal, pine, plum; soften the effect by topping with a taupe eye shadow

Mascara

Brown, black or pine

Blush

Salmon or bronzing powder as blush

Lipstick

Terracotta, mahogany or tomato red to warm up your look; soft plum or claret for a cooler look

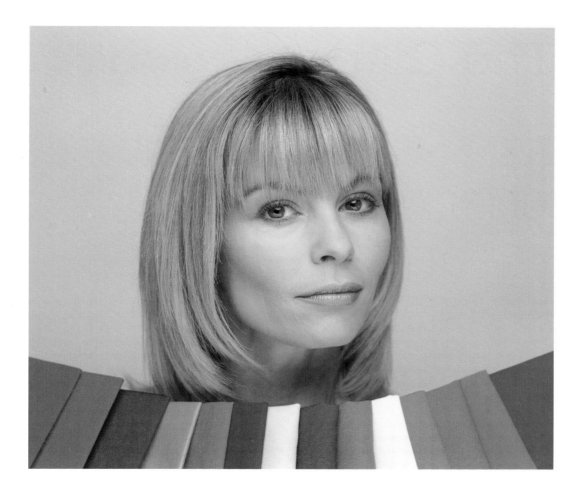

Colours to wear

Plenty of choice and variety awaits the woman with soft colouring, from soft white and ivory instead of pure white, to charcoal, taupe or soft navy instead of black.

Your colours should never be bright: think 'subdued'. Soft rose pinks or salmons, as well as matte or soft reds, are lovely alone or when teamed with neutral colours. Rich spruce, forest or jade greens are a must for the soft wardrobe, along with muted blues such as teal or periwinkle. Violets, purples and aubergines are lovely with navy or chocolate.

The Clear Wardrobe

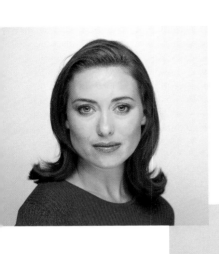

Successful

Jewel tones are your best bets for work or play. Think vibrant, striking. Your natural colouring deserves nothing less.

Least successful

Why just look okay, like this, when you could look terrific instead?

Overall impression

Bright and contrasting

Color Me Beautiful seasons

Clear Spring, Clear Winter

Famous examples

Courtney Cox, Princess Caroline of Monaco, Oprah Winfrey

Goals

To complement your bright look with clear colours that are vibrant

Helpful hints

Avoid greyed-down shades on their own. Contrast light colours with dark ones and add bright colours to liven up neutrals

Make-up advice

Eyes

Navy, grey, plum, pine; ivory, apricot or soft pink highlighter

Brows

Cocoa or taupe to blend with your own

Liner

Black, navy, grey, plum, spruce

Mascara

Black, navy or pine

Blush

Hot pink or clear salmon; soft red when wearing red lipstick

Lipstick

Hot pink for a cool look; coral for a warm look; true red

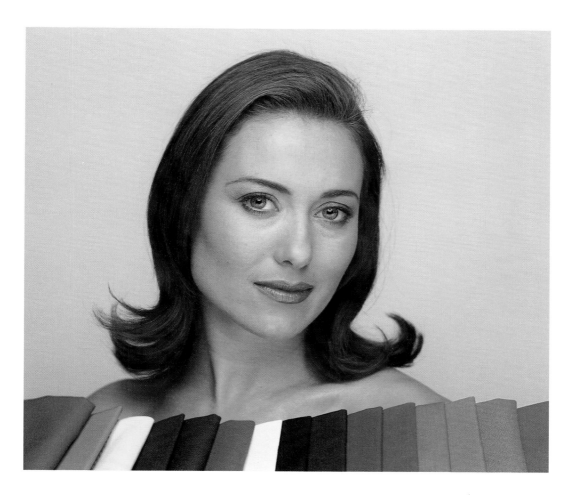

Colours to wear

Wear your wonderful wardrobe in combination or solid blocks. Any of these colours can rescue items in your wardrobe that are not up to scratch colourwise.

Pure or soft whites are preferable to creamy shades. Your neutrals are rich and inky, from jet black and navy to charcoal and black-brown.

Hot pink should be great, but if you are pushing your colouring warmer (such as with hair colour), add mango, coral and clear salmon shades. Your best red is scarlet. Keep blues rich like sapphire, greens bright like emerald and yellow as sparkling as topaz.

Change Your
Co

ouring

A dramatic change to your natural colouring can result in a personality change as well. I have done several TV programmes on the subject and heard testimonials from natural brunettes who, 'born again' as blonde, took on completely different personality and behavioural traits.

'As a brunette, I never felt sexy,' confessed one bleached convert, who had lovely features and a terrific figure. 'As a blonde, I feel I can move differently and flirt quite openly, like I always wanted to but felt foolish doing as a brunette.'

I don't buy the notion that gentlemen necessarily prefer blondes. Perhaps thirty years ago, with Marilyn mania at its height, blondes did have more fun. But a woman of any colouring can be, and should feel, attractive. Pint-size siren Winona Ryder, a natural blonde, dyes her hair dark because she 'feels like a brunette'. The desire for opposite colouring can apply to any woman, blonde, brunette, redhead or white-haired.

If your colouring affects how you feel about yourself and you want a change, then go for it! This chapter gives you guidelines for choosing the best options, taking into account your natural colouring, age and the amount of hassle you are prepared put up with to maintain your new look.

Read through the options for your natural colouring. If in any doubt, seek the advice of a good colourist, who should be delighted to give advice before doing any work. Bring in pictures of the colour or effects you would like to achieve and hear what's involved and the amount of maintenance required. Allow the colourist to put together the right formulation to achieve *your* desired result. If you want to discuss the implications for your wardrobe and make-up before or after you colour your hair (this is critical), please get in touch with us (see page 191).

The safe option: Go with nature

Here's a great example of what can happen when you defy Mother Nature. Stunning actress Louise Lombard, not a natural blonde, was recently pressured to totally revamp herself. What motivates the superstars to radically alter their natural looks is generally a pitch for much-needed publicity rather than an honest attempt to make more of their own beauty. Lombard's natural celtic colouring – jet hair, piercing blue eyes and porcelain skin – is almost negated by the peroxide bleach job. Considering her youth and the skill of a top colourist and make-up artist, Lombard loses her stunning impact by attempting a make-over so diametrically opposed to her own colouring.

As you will read in this chapter, all women have myriad options to enhance or change their looks. A new hair colour can revitalize your image. But the wrong hair colour can make you look ill or years older. Who needs that?

The safest option is always to go with nature by deepening or highlighting, warming up or cooling down your locks, according to your own genetic chemistry. In the following sections, you will see guidelines for pushing your colouring to look more dramatic, healthier, younger or softer within the limits of what will compliment your skin and eyes.

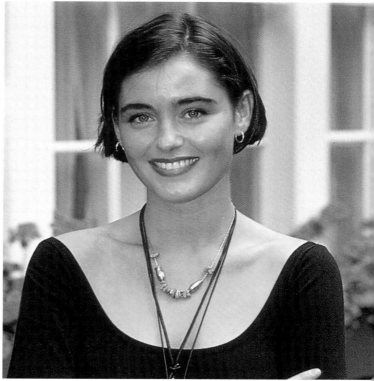

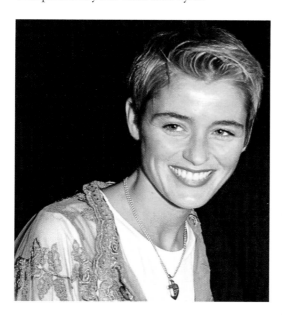

Colouring Options

Vegetable dyes or rinses: These use natural plant and vegetable pigments to coat the hair and therefore provide temporary colour (which gradually fades over six to eight shampoos). The one exception is henna, which stains the hair permanently. On dark hair, henna will give a warm, auburn effect; light hair, henna turns

strawberry blonde, or worse – orange. Unlike vegetable shampoos, henna takes up to two hours to apply and process.

Temporary colour: Great as a pick-me-up for your natural hair colour or to remove brassy tones from white or blonde hair. Temporary treatments also provide a boost between applications of more permanent treatments. These take just a couple of minutes to apply and come in the form of shampoo, mousse or setting lotion. The colour just sticks to the outside cuticle of the hair and washes out after shampooing.

Semi-permanent colour: A bit more effort is required here as these liquids, creams and mousses take about half an hour to apply and process. They darken hair by adding tone but will not lighten hair. The colour goes deeper into the hair shaft than with temporary colour and stays through six to eight shampoos, fading gradually. Semi-permanents are good for helping a modest amount of grey hair blend more naturally into your natural colour. Longer-lasting formulas of semi-permanents use peroxide to help the colour penetrate deeper into the hair follicle: these can be effective for up to twelve shampoos.

Permanent colour: These take about 45 minutes to apply and process, and require a firm commitment as they don't fade out, but grow out. Tints are for lightening, darkening or enriching colour.

Taking Care of Coloured Hair

✦ Protect for the first 3 days after treatment: no sun or swimming.

✦ Use a shampoo and conditioner specially for coloured/treated hair. They help to lock the colour into the hair follicles, which means the colour will last longer, as well as reinforcing the hair's condition after treatment.

✦ Let the hair dry naturally as often as possible, or use the hairdryer on a cool setting.

✦ In the sun, protect your hair by using special shampoos, gels and oils with sunblocks (UVB filters).

A Change of Colour

JANE Like too many natural redheads, Jane hates her colouring. She's been a brunette and a blonde and avoids going anywhere near a colour described as strawberry, copper or auburn.

With about 25 per cent of her hair now grey, Jane had been advised to try ash blonde to disguise it. Sure, her hair was pretty. But against her warm, freckled skin, it made her look in serious need of a shot of Vitamin B12. When your natural colouring is so definitely warm, it is essential to keep

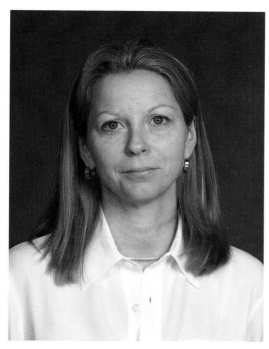

consider its effect on your skin tone and your make-up. If in doubt about a new direction, try what worked for Jane by having a new, experimental shade woven in as a trial for a new look. Next time you might be ready to go even further. Jane's considering going ginger!

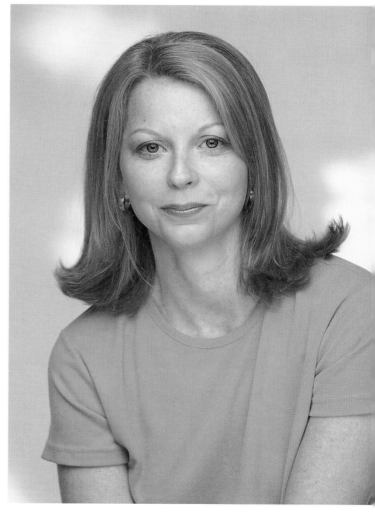

the undertone of any new choice golden rather than ash.

Defying her warm skin tone and soft blue eyes, Jane wore either pinky-toned make-up or flat, neutral browns – neither of which enhance her. Pink tones are too cool and the neutral browns too muted for her natural colouring.

As Jane was reluctant to go the full copper-red route, she took Wella's advice and let them weave in some copper strands among the blonde streaks to warm her up and make more of her skin tone. Jane valued this measured approach to testing a new colour, and followed our advice for warmer make-up and wardrobe colours.

When selecting a shade of blonde,

Deep Colouring

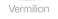

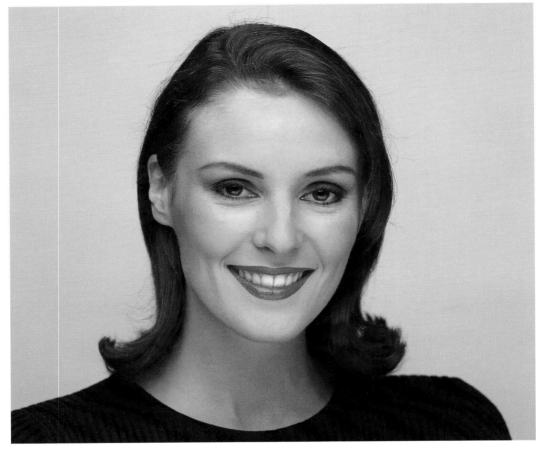

Dark eyes; dark hair

Women with brunette, chestnut, deep auburn or black hair who were never blonde (after the age of five) should avoid blonde highlights until later in life, unless after a striking, obviously artificial effect, such as a black or Japanese woman with blonde hair.

Call me old-fashioned, but I think that blonde hair on a woman over thirty-five with obviously deep colour is a little sad. Up until the menopause, women with deep colouring have strong skin tone, rich eyebrows and eye colour and only look like they are wearing a wig if they dye their hair blonde.

Highlights

As Caucasian women age, their skin tone and eye colour softens and lighter highlights in grey and chestnut hair become possible. The hair should now almost be mousy, no longer the rich chestnut or black it once was. Beautiful salt 'n' pepper hair can be conditioned with a semi-permanent rinse which gives shine to normally dull white strands and deepens the dark strands.

Make-up tips: If you are naturally going lighter, adapt your make-up colours from rich burgundy, berry or plum tones to softer shades. If you love wearing red, soften down the lipstick with a natural-colour lip pencil underneath. Use a neutral, warm blush, avoiding anything too muddy, dark or bright.

Highlights make your face look warmer and softer, so grey and brown shadows will be better neutrals than black and navy. Use peach highlighters.

Wardrobe tips: You will discover that black, dark brown or navy near the face is too harsh. See the Soft Wardrobe ideas on pages 98–99 to get a feel for for your direction. Avoid bold contrasts in prints, and opt for blended and monochromatic effects.

Auburn Rinse, Warm Lowlights

Going warmer can look wonderful on women with deep colouring. Try a henna treatment or a semi-auburn, bronze or copper rinse. Real drama queens can head straight for a flaming copper tint. Lowlights will have a brightening as well as a warming effect, especially on brown hair.

Make-up tips: For lipsticks, going 'warmer' means you should avoid pinks, fuchsias or burgundy tones. Red will be wonderful, as will terracotta, mahogany, salmon and peach. Make use of brown, olive and aubergine in your eyeshadows, with a melon or apricot highlighter. Steer clear of grey or blue shadows. Salmon pink blush is best.

Wardrobe tips:

As with your make-up, avoid pinks unless salmon or coral; softer versions are more flattering than bright ones. All greens will work – moss, jade and olive to forest green. Experiment with entirely new colour combinations: try rust and aubergine or mustard with tomato red.

Plum Tones

Plum or burgundy colourings make you and your skin look 'cooler'. Also try dramatic deep damson or violet.

Make-up tips: Berry, plum, red and hot pink will be your most effective lipsticks. Avoid tan or brown lipsticks, which can look muddy against your cool mane. In eyeshadow, grey, navy and plum will be most striking; for highlighter, use pink or champagne. Rose or pink blushes complete the effect.

Wardrobe tips: Look at the Deep Wardrobe (pages 92–93) and the Cool Wardrobe (pages 94–95) to see how you can blend the palettes for best effect. Blues, pinks, greys and purples will be particularly stunning on you now. Avoid warm colours like rust, yellow, beiges and browns (except black-brown).

Light Colouring

GOLDEN HIGHLIGHTS

Beige Doré

Savannah Gold

Light Blonde

GOING RED

Indian Gold

Soft Irish Copper

Sierra Gold

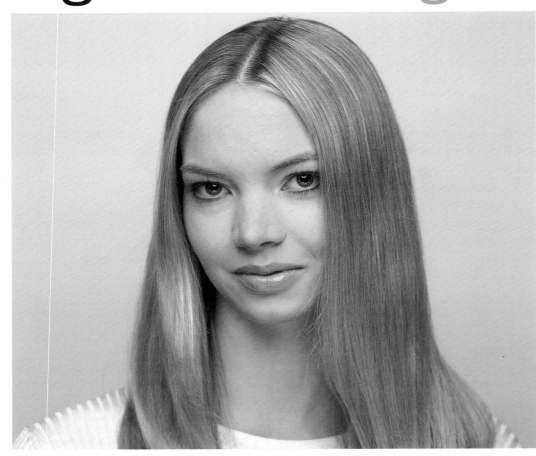

Light hair; light eyes

You probably shouldn't consider going dark unless you don't mind looking like you're wearing a wig. The maintenance of dark hair also requires regular root treatment, eyebrow- and lash-tinting for best effect. Warming-up or highlighting your hair will be your best options.

Golden Highlights

To look like an angel, give yourself a halo. Hold up clumps of hair tints near your face (without any, or just 'natural', make-up) and see which looks healthiest. Try two or three different shades of blonde for a more natural, sun-kissed result; for example, a light natural blonde mixed with strands of golden blonde and a soft copper gold.

Make-up tips: As you are already fair, your make-up won't need any adjusting, provided you are already wearing the best colours (see pages 90–91). In lipstick, keep it soft and light, never too dark. Rather than brighten your lipstick, try lip gloss over a natural pencil. Soft brown or grey shadows are best, or blue-grey if your eyes are blue. Use a lemon or peachy-pink highlighter. Avoid black mascara, which is too harsh, in favour of a medium brown. A soft pink blush is your best.

Wardrobe tips: Camel will become your most elegant neutral colour, with the greys looking less exciting the more golden you go. If you insist on wearing black, show as much flesh between your face and the neckline as possible. Avoid white in favour of ivory; bold prints are a no-go area.

Going Red

Blondes who have naturally warm skin (for example, some freckles) can often look terrific as redheads. If in doubt, take it a step at a time by trying strawberry, soft copper or golden blonde before you dive head first into carrot!

Make-up tips: Moving into a warmer direction requires your make-up to be less rosy pink and more creamy and peachy. The best lipsticks will be corals and salmon (or flaming orange for evening). Any brown will be your best shadow, but if your eyes are blue, try grey. Highlighters can be peachy pink or melon. Avoid rosy or brown blushes in favour of light, warm pink.

Wardrobe tips: Greys look less stunning now than camels, blondes and warm golds as your best neutrals. Some warm browns and greens can be muddy – your best ones will be clear and bright. All your pinks need to have a warm undertone (orange or yellow base) rather than be too icy or blue pink.

Cool Colouring

HIGHLIGHTS

Champagne

Medium Blonde

Dark Brown

DEEPENING RINSE/ LOWLIGHTS

Alizarin

Carmine

Jet Black

BLUE TONES

Purple Rain

Blue Moon

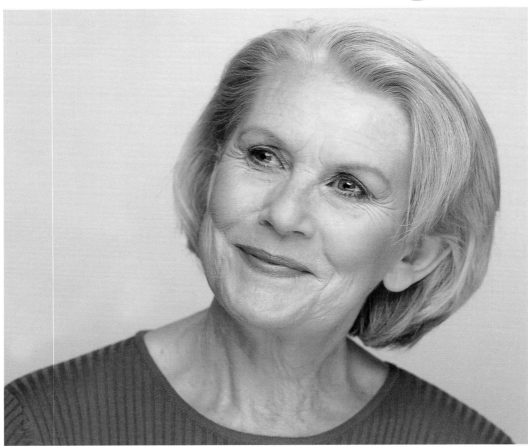

Ash-brown, grey or white hair; blue or brown eyes

Because of your striking looks you have several good choices for changing your colouring with dramatic effect. If you don't want to worry friends about your health, you are wise to avoid going red or auburn, which will fight too much with your natural colouring.

Highlights

With highlights, you are opting to lighten your overall colouring. As your skin and eyes are 'cool', try ash lights rather than very golden ones for best effect. You can mix highlights, too: try a light ash and a soft pearl with a light neutral blonde.

Make-up tips: You won't have to make any adjustments from your usual palette of rosy pink, plum and red lipsticks (avoiding brown tones altogether). In eyeshadows, try cocoa-brown or grey with pale pink or champagne highlighter. For blush, soft plum or dusty rose are best.

Wardrobe tips: Be careful not to go deeper or brighter than your cool palette of colours (see the Cool Wardrobe ideas on pages 94–95). Very stark contrasts like black and white or bold prints are inadvisable.

Deepening Rinse or Lowlights

Enriching your hair will result in adding some warmth to your colouring. This can look wonderful provided you stop short of going too copper or very golden. Try burgundy, damson or heather tones.

Make-up tips: A warmer mane will conflict with very cool (that is, pink) make-up. Push your pinks into pinky-browns. Eyeshadows should be kept neutral, with no hint of blue or green, in favour of cocoa-browns, greys or plums, complemented with a peachy-pink highlighter. The best blush will be the most natural, almost indiscernible, colour.

Wardrobe tips: Deepening your colouring means that you can get away with black more easily than before. If the lowlights really come up warm, try using brown with your pinks for an elegant new look. The pale blues won't be as interesting as teal and turquoise. A very dark navy may not be as flattering as before, so use charcoal grey instead. Look at the Soft Wardrobe ideas on pages 98–99, along with your own Cool Wardrobe on pages 94–95, and you will see many possibilities for harmonizing your wardrobe with your new hair colour.

Blue, Violet or Pink Rinses

Cool chicks with white hair often like to experiment with a rinse. Some brave over-sixties have led the way for spunky punks by adopting quite unnatural but fun ways to perk up their white hair. You do need quite a personality to carry off a pink or violet crop!

Imagine the effects of adding a bold colour to a pot of white paint. The same thing will happen when you try a strong hair colour on yourself: the result will be a pastel version of the tint. For example, an orange rinse creates an apricot crop, while purple would give you a lilac mane. What fun!

Make-up tips: These tones are all cool, so your make-up needn't change from the rosy pinks and plums for lipsticks; soft cocoa and grey with a little pink for eyeshadow, and pinky blush.

Wardrobe tips: As with your make-up, your Cool Wardrobe (pages 94–95) will complement any cool rinse or tint. Rather than be concerned about colour, be sure your style isn't too staid for your flamboyant hair.

Warm Colouring

HIGHLIGHTS

Beige Doré

Savannah Gold

Indian Gold

LOWLIGHTS

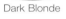

Dark Blonde

Havannah

Irish Chestnut

EVEN REDDER

Venetian Red

Indian Copper

Soft Irish Copper

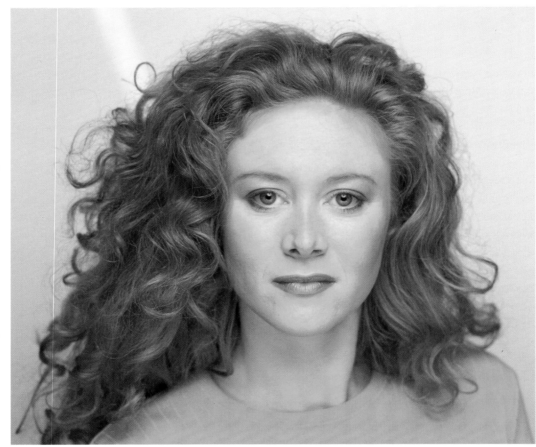

Golden blonde, strawberry, red, warm brown hair; green, blue, topaz eyes

You have a variety of options for colouring your hair, with the best advice never to go much darker or cooler (such as ash blonde) than you are already. The result of either choice would be that you look seriously unwell. Best bets include soft copper blondes, copper golds or golden sandy tints.

Change Your Colouring ● 115

Highlights

If you want to be blonde, go golden, never ash blonde. This is especially good to consider when you start going grey or white, as you want to retain warmth in your hair for as long as possible to look your best. Try a golden sand, oyster beige or golden blonde for best results.

Make-up tips: Going blonde from redder hair means steering clear of very brown lipstick and blushes. You will look brighter in warm pinks for both. For eyeshadows, smoky teals, grey or cocoa-brown are lovely, especially teamed with peach highlighters.

Wardrobe tips: Little needs to change with your wardrobe. Your skin tone will never be complemented by hot pinks, so keep to the peaches and apricots. Camel remains your best neutral (over navy, grey and black). Ivory, of course, will still be more flattering than white. Compare the Light Wardrobe ideas on pages 90–91 with your own Warm Wardrobe on pages 96–97 to see how you might best integrate your colours.

Lowlights

Lowlights will add depth, tone and zip. If you want a subtle effect, try dark golden blonde. For more sparkle, go for deep copper golds or even a flame-red or claret.

Make-up tips: As you are brightening your look, avoid dull browns, especially in your lipsticks and blushes. Lift your new colouring by adding a salmon blush and a touch of deep peach to the centre of your lips (perhaps over a terracotta base). Eyeshadows can remain browns or soft grey and peach.

Wardrobe tips: No changes are needed, only consider slightly brighter tones or fabrics than the usual matt or nubby textures so lovely on deeper auburn types.

Go Even Redder

If your skin is fair and your eyes are bright, why not go copper or claret-red for a flaming effect on the world? Try a rich auburn tint or rinse if your eyes are brown or green. If you have blue eyes, choose a rinse or tint that has a brightening not a dulling effect, such as a flaming red.

Make-up tips: No change from your usual warm colours, though you might now be brave enough to try an orange lipstick. Golden touches for the evening in your eyeshadow, lipstick or blush will have a devastating effect.

Wardrobe tips: Now every colour in your palette will be magic. With added drama in your hair, make sure your style is equally dramatic.

Clear Colouring

HIGHLIGHTS

Dark Blonde

Medium Blonde

Light Brown

GOING DEEPER

Jet Black

Dark Brown

Carmine

WARM RINSES

Alizarin

COOL RINSES

Purple Rain

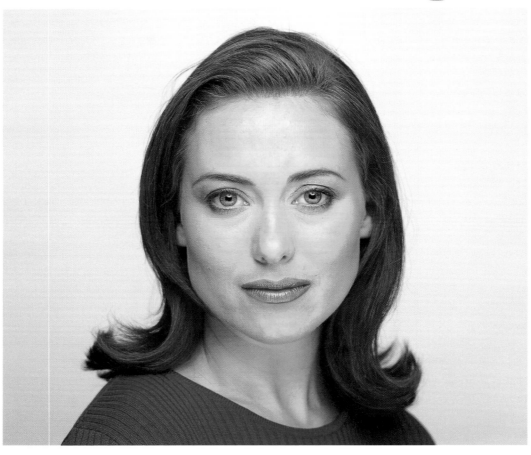

Medium to dark brown, black or salt 'n' pepper hair; bright blue, green, hazel or black-brown eyes

Highlights

Going lighter is worth a think if you start to go grey. Before the signs of any grey, however, as you were probably never a natural blonde, highlights might look artificial on you and take away the drama of your brilliant colouring.

Some temporary or semi-permanent colours can help to brighten up white strands and add depth to your natural colour. The added value will be the boost of shine to the usual dull finish of white and grey hair.

Make-up tips: The results of going lighter will mean that your look will soften and be warmer (so avoid ash highlights in favour of soft, golden tones). Your make-up, therefore, requires a major overhaul.

Out goes red or any bright lipstick in favour of colours softened with a natural-colour lip pencil underneath. Shadows now must be neutral and always matt (even for evening). Blush should be a salmon pink.

Wardrobe tips: As with your make-up, it's overhaul time in the wardrobe if you lighten your hair. Avoid strong contrasts like black and red or royal blue and white in favour of blended colours like pewter and purple or navy and brown. Compare the Soft Wardrobe ideas on pages 98–99 with your current Clear Wardrobe on pages 100–101 to see the contrast. Don't go lighter on impulse. Reflect on the consequences before you plunge.

Going Deeper

If you are in search of a drop-dead Snow White look, give this a go. Beware if you are over thirty-five, as an all-over colour tint can be aging on your face. Discuss with your colourist how to keep the depth without adding harshness by mixing tones to suit you.

Make-up tips: Red will be your winner lipstick for day or night. Keep your eyes as bright as your overall look with rich charcoal eyeshadow set against the palest pink, lilac or champagne highlighter. Your blush can be a warm pink or even a red-pink.

Wardrobe tips: For best effect, wear solid colours or just two colours together. Forget prints except for black or navy and white. Never wear anything beige.

Warm (Auburn) or Cool (Burgundy) Rinses and Tints

Give either a try, aware that you need to make wardrobe and make-up adjustments. The advice is the same as for Deep Colouring (see page 109).

Soft Colouring

DEEPENING RINSE

Sahara Gold

Dark Blonde

Persimmon

HIGHLIGHTS

Champagne (cool)

Beige Doré (warm)

GOING RED

Warm Heather

Sierra Gold

Indian Bronze

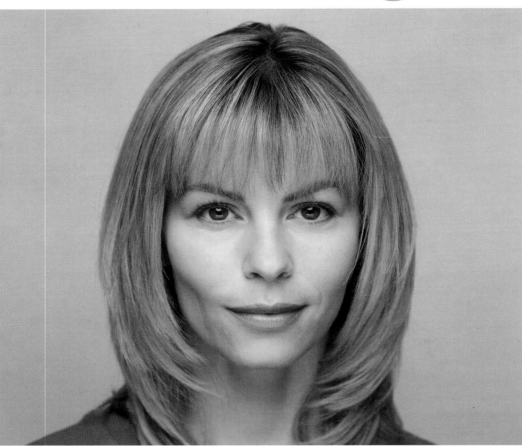

Dark blonde, medium/mousy brown hair; brown, hazel or blue-grey eyes

Your natural colouring lends itself best to experimenting with hair colour because your naturally 'neutral' base can be taken successfully in a variety of directions.

A Deepening Rinse or Tint

By strengthening your hair colour, say with a chestnut or bronze rinse, you add both depth and warmth to your hair. Test strands to see if a warmer tone is flattering on your skin, or whether you are better in a richer, more neutral, deep brown.

Make-up tips: Going deeper may accentuate natural circles and lines around the eyes. If you don't use concealer, it's probably time you did. Your eyes will now take on more definition and will suit smoky effects well. Rather than using very dark colours, try building more depth by blending a few soft tones together, such as grey and plum or cocoa and olive.

Test whether a cooler pink or warm peach is the better highlighter on you now. Lipsticks can go richer into mahogany and berry tones and are best kept matt, not glossy. Red remains a no-go zone unless you ground it with a natural-colour lip pencil underneath.

Wardrobe tips: Your wardrobe now requires more depth, and black will be far more interesting than when you were your natural mousy self. Compare the Deep Wardrobe on pages 92–93 with your own Soft Wardrobe on pages 98–99 to consider how to blend the two. Don't go brighter in your clothes, just richer.

Highlights

Lightening your hair can make you look much more alive. Test sample patches against your skin to see whether a light golden blonde or light ash blonde would be better.

Make-up tips: The key is to keep it soft and neutral. The undertone will be cool if you choose

ash blonde highlights, or warm if you go golden. See Cool Colouring (page 112) or Warm Colouring (page 114).

Wardrobe tips: Highlighting your hair will have no impact on your wardrobe. Continue to enjoy your colours.

Going Red: Copper or Auburn

Here's a great option, especially for soft types with brown or hazel eyes. When you are over forty, lowlights might be more flattering and give you the added warmth that you want. A rich auburn can be terrific, especially if your eyes are a strong colour. If your eyebrows are light, consider tinting them as well. Highlights of warm copper mixed with lowlights of a deep auburn chestnut are particularly attractive.

Make-up tips: Blues or greys will be dreadful on you. Opt now for warm brown, sage or aubergine,

with pale peach highlighter. Your blush and lipstick should be terracotta or cinnamon. When wearing red, make sure it is warm (orange base) not cool (blue base).

Wardrobe tips: You've been longing for some drama, so complete the look in your clothes as well. Team any wishy-washy neutrals with a vivid blast of colour from the warm palette (see the Warm Wardrobe ideas on page 97), which you can blend with your own Soft Wardrobe (page 99).

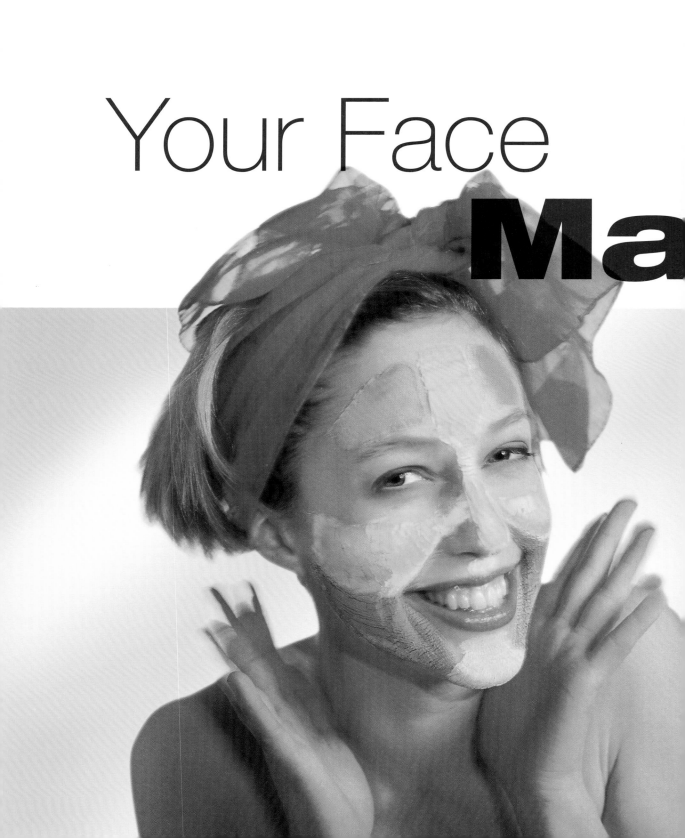

Your Face

Ma

keover

The impact of a great outfit or new hairstyle can be lost if you don't look well groomed with make-up. The right make-up can be quite undetectable and very natural, or it can pull out all the stops and create drama to match an equally dramatic outfit. The choice is yours.

What isn't optional, however, is going without – aside from when you are playing sports, hanging out at home or in the garden, or just telling the world you've got to get off for a while.

This book is all about image and how you can make the most of your natural beauty. If you are under twenty and quite flawless, surely you will look sweet without make-up. But maybe you are tired of 'sweet' and now want to look serious or seriously sexy. Well, girl, make-up is the answer.

Your make-up will look more luminous, and expensive, if you apply it to a properly cleansed and treated face. The beauty columns bombard us with new products and ideas to try. The right routine depends on your own skin, your lifestyle and how much you want to spend on products. You can look wonderful by spending a little time but not much money if you want. You can also do more harm than good to your skin by using too many or the wrong products.

The condition of your skin is determined by your genes, your diet and exercise, the environment and your age. Your genetic chemistry is a given, but we can deal with the other factors. What you eat (and drink) is all-important, so let's look at that first.

Diet

Care for your skin should begin on the inside. No amount of treatment products will counteract the effects of too many toxins in your diet, insufficient water, a lack of essential nutrients, smoking, and so on. Unless you eat a good, well-balanced diet, you need to take supplements to get the nutrients that you need for good skin tone.

Essential Nutrients for Your Skin

Iron: Along with calcium, this is the major dietary deficiency in women. It needs some vitamin C, copper, cobalt or manganese to be assimilated. If you are a heavy coffee or tea drinker, you are inhibiting the natural absorption of iron from the food you eat.

Food sources of iron include liver and kidney, red meat, egg yolks, oily fish, oysters, nuts, beans and lentils, green leafy vegetables, asparagus, oatmeal, dried peaches, molasses and chocolate.

If these foods are lacking in your diet, you should take a supplement in the form of a multivitamin. A blood test will confirm the level of deficiency and whether you need a stronger dose of iron. In addition to poor skin, iron deficiency is manifest by general fatigue and vulnerability to colds and viruses.

Sulphur: This is often used topically (that is, applied externally to the affected area) in the treatment of skin conditions, and is essential in your diet for healthy hair, skin and nails. Provided you have protein in your diet you will be getting the sulphur required for healthy skin.

Food sources of sulphur include lean beef, beans, fish, eggs and cabbage.

PABA (Para-aminobenzoic acid): PABA helps to minimize wrinkles and keep the skin healthy. Eczema can result from a serious deficiency of PABA. If your diet is rich in B vitamins, you will be getting what is needed. If not, consider a B-complex supplement.

Food sources of PABA include brewer's yeast, Marmite, liver, kidney, whole grains, wheatgerm and molasses.

Vitamin C: The star antioxidant, and a prime vitamin not only for good health but also for cell regeneration and the absorption of iron. Smokers should consider taking 1000mg daily to get additional help in absorbing the nutrients from their diet, something which smoking inhibits.

Food sources of vitamin C include fruits (especially citrus), green and leafy vegetables, tomatoes, potatoes and peppers.

Your Skin Type

Every major department store is equipped with microscopes, videos and other special gear to analyse your skin. It is depressing stuff to see your skin magnified a thousand times, even if you are only twenty-five – all those cracks and signs of damage. The important thing, however, is how oily or dry your skin is.

You probably have an idea of your skin type. Oily skin gets irritatingly shiny, while dry skin feels itchy and uncomfortable if not moisturized properly. If it isn't definitely either one, you probably have combination skin. A way to find out which type of skin you have is to wash your face with your usual cleanser, then leave it without any moisturizer for thirty minutes. If within ten minutes you feel some tightness, your skin is dry. If you wipe a tissue over your nose and chin after thirty minutes and there is some surface oil, then your skin is oily. Otherwise, you probably have combination skin, with an oilier T-zone (forehead, nose and chin) and some dryness or normal skin elsewhere.

Your skin can and does change, not just with age but with the time of year and with your environment, both indoors and out of doors. Women who work in offices with centrally controlled air systems tend to develop dry skin conditions because of the lack of moisture in the air. Outside, exposure to either sun or wind will dry out the oiliest of skins and wreak havoc with combination and drier skin types.

Hence, you need to watch your skin throughout the year and give it the nourishment (both in what you eat and in what you apply to it) that it needs to remain in peak condition.

SWEAT 'N' GLO

Nothing clears the skin better than a good workout. Any aerobic activity that gets the heart and blood pumping and the sweat flowing helps to flush out the toxins lurking underneath the skin. Clogged pores and blackheads are purged more easily after a good workout.

Immediately after exercise you will look hot, bothered and blotchy. Have a shower, cool down and you will be glowing within 30 minutes.

The right stuff: cleanse, tone and moisturize

All skins benefit from a twice-daily routine. In the morning your face is covered with dead cells, pushed off by the new cells produced underneath. If you apply make-up directly over dead skin you will, as you might expect, look blotchier than you need. So always be sure to cleanse well, to follow up with a non-alcohol toner to remove any traces of dead skin, oil and cleanser, and then to moisturize. Very oily skins can add an extra wipe of witch hazel to act as an antiseptic over problem areas. Here is how to treat the three main skin types.

Dry Skin

Protection and moisturizing are the keys. Avoid cleansers containing 'detergents', such as surfactants, no matter how mild they are alleged to be, because they may strip what little natural oil you have in your skin. Opt instead for mild, cream cleansers made with as many natural ingredients as possible. Essential oils such as camomile and lavender are particularly good on dry skins, so look for cleansers that contain these.

Massage cleanser gently all over your face to remove make-up. Wipe away cleanser, grime and make-up with moistened cottonwool pads. Repeat a second time, particularly if you are clearing off a full face of make-up. Alternatively, patting off cleanser with a warm, wet flannel will give you a fresh and clean sensation while adding some welcome water back into the surface of the skin.

A protective moisturize in the morning and at night will prevent the skin from becoming dehydrated and flaky. The drier the skin, the richer the cream you should use, especially at night when the skin works hard regenerating cells. Indeed, a rich night cream can provide hydration and oil enrichment that would be too heavy under make-up during the day.

Combination Skin

Follow the cleansing advice for drier, more delicate skin types in the winter, and switch to a gel or facial foam made of mild detergent in the summer if your skin feels grubbier then. Water-soluble gels are good for combination and oily skin types and restore moisture to the skin in the process.

Use moisturizer on the forehead, cheeks and neck and gently wipe off any excess that hasn't been absorbed within five minutes. So, cleanse, tone and moisturize first thing in the morning, then get on to other tasks (having a cup of tea, making the bed, getting dressed) before checking to see that all the moisturizer has gone in. Your make-up will look better and last longer during the day if you don't apply it over an excess of moisturizing lotion.

Oily Skin

Your priority is cleansing, to unblock pores and keep trouble (namely spots) at bay. Cleansing creams will make your skin more greasy, so opt for a gel or foam cleanser of an alkaline solution (one that will restore the skin's PH balance).

Facial scrubs are good to use as an evening cleanser but don't use them every day, and only use them during a time when your sebaceous (oil-producing) glands seem to be in overdrive. Rather than rip away at your skin with a flannel, use your fingers to gently work in the scrubs to lift make-up and impurities.

A light moisturizing cream is an important final step – to keep moisture in the skin and pollutants out – but avoid using any over the T-zone or areas with already enlarged pores and spots.

Learn the Lingo

AHAs (Alpha-hydroxy acids) Natural acids found in fruit, sugar and milk, which loosen dead cells so that the skin appears fresher. Creams containing AHAs have a mild exfoliating effect, smoothing the skin while boosting cellular action.

Antioxidants These are wonder vitamins such as A, C and E, which attract and stabilize free radicals (molecules in the body and on the skin upset by pollution, smoking and sunlight).

Ceramides Fatty lipids present in the skin, which provide a natural moisture barrier. Products containing synthetic ceramides help strengthen this barrier, bond skin cells and plump up the skin.

Collagen A protein connecting tissue in the dermis (two layers beneath the surface) that gives the skin its strength.

Elastin Along with collagen in the dermis, this protein gives smoothness to the skin. Products containing elastin help the skin appear smoother.

Liposomes Tiny spheres of water and fat that move ingredients to where the skin needs them.

Moisture boosters These are more than simple moisturizers as they include a super-duper hydrating agent called hyaluronic acid. Good for counteracting dryness, they trap moisture in the tissues.

SPF or sun protection factor A scale of how effectively sunscreen products protect the skin from UVB rays. For example, if your skin takes just ten minutes to burn in the sun, an SPF 15 cream will give you protection for fifteen times longer – so you could stay out in the sun for two and a half hours (150 minutes) before starting to sizzle.

Skin firmers Made up of active ingredients such as botanical extracts that help to tighten superficial skin layers. There is no proof, despite claims, that skin firmers restore collagen and elastin.

Vitamin moisture creams These use the antioxidant properties of Vitamin E to prevent free radicals doing their damage, or the natural moisture-enhancing properties of Vitamin A.

Skin-Care Essentials for Mid-Lifers

AHA cream With cell renewal slowing down, sloughing off dead cells, which can make the skin look dull, is key. But exfoliants are too rough for your skin, now that it is thinner than it once was. An AHA cream will naturally exfoliate without damaging the skin. Once converted you won't want to be without it.

Cleansers and toners Only the most gentle cleansers will do. Use those cleansing minutes to massage the skin, lifting off dead cells along with make-up and pollution. Toners must be alcohol-free.

Anti-ageing creams Recent medical research proves that some do, indeed, plump up the skin and reduce the appearance of wrinkles. If you get hooked on them, be prepared to do without a night on the town once a month 'cause these wonder creams don't come cheap.

Eye creams/gels Even a thirty-year-old knows just how delicate the tissue around the eye becomes. Preserve this delicate skin with a good cream or gel specially for the eye area. Avoid rich night creams here, as they can make this fine skin sag.

Masks Opt for a moisturizing mask once a week to give the skin an extra boost, not to mention giving you an extra treat.

Night cream Okay, your face doesn't know the time of day, but applying a richer moisturizer while you sleep gives the skin an extra dose of much-needed hydration. There are special solutions for the face, neck, hands and body should your budget extend that far. At the minimum, invest in your face.

Make-Up and
Beauty Equipment

Here is all that you need to know about make-up, starting with the essential gear you need.

Dressing Table Gear
Essentials:

- Foundation and sponge
- Concealer
- Loose, translucent powder with puff and large brush
- Eyeshadows and three key brushes (long handles)
- Blush and blush brush

- Tweezers
- Kohl pencil eyeliners
- Mascara and comb/brush combo
- Lip pencil
- Three lipsticks to coordinate with your whole wardrobe, including your best red
- Pencil sharpener

Optional extras:

- Eyelash curler
- Eyebrow pencil (brown shadow can do the job)

- Bronzing powder
- Lip gloss
- White kohl pencil

Make-Up Bag Gear

How much you carry around in your handbag for touch-ups will depend on your lifestyle and the demands on you to look polished throughout the day. Women who leave home early and might need to transform themselves for the evening without the luxury of a pit-stop at home will need the following:

- Powder foundation or pressed powder: for more coverage, opt for the former
- A combination blush and eyeshadow compact for a quick touch-up

- A charcoal eyeliner can deepen any colour you might have used earlier and make your lashes look even thicker
- Mascara

✦ Lip pencil

✦ Gloss or lipstick

✦ Small bottle of perfume

Hygiene Pays

Keep your make-up gear clean to avoid spreading bacteria and infection. Clean kit will last longer and give you better value for money. Factor in several years of potential use for brushes, months for powder puffs and weeks for sponges.

Make-up sponges should be washed out after every use. Allow to air dry. Compact sponges/puffs need a weekly wash if used daily. Throw sponges and puffs into the washing machine in an old pair of tights every few weeks for a good, thorough wash.

Rinse your brushes every ten days if you use them daily. Fill the basin up with warm water and a little shampoo and swirl the brush heads around. Rinse. Lip brushes require a swipe across a bar of soap and a good squeeze to get rid of all product. Shape the brush after rinsing and leave to air dry.

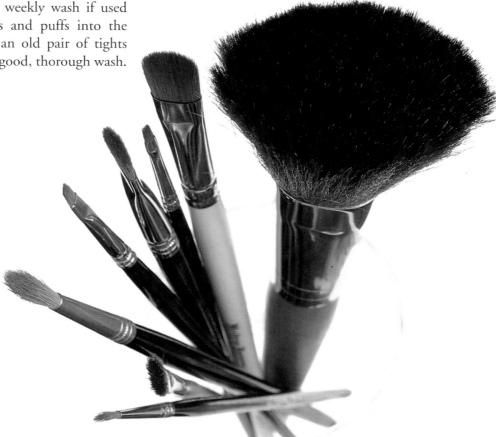

Foundation

Go with nature. The worst mistake in choosing foundation is to pick a colour that is very different from your natural skin tone. You might wish to have rosier skin or to look more tanned, but trying to create that effect with your foundation won't work. The wrong-coloured foundation makes you look either unwell or dirty.

If you are shopping for new foundation,

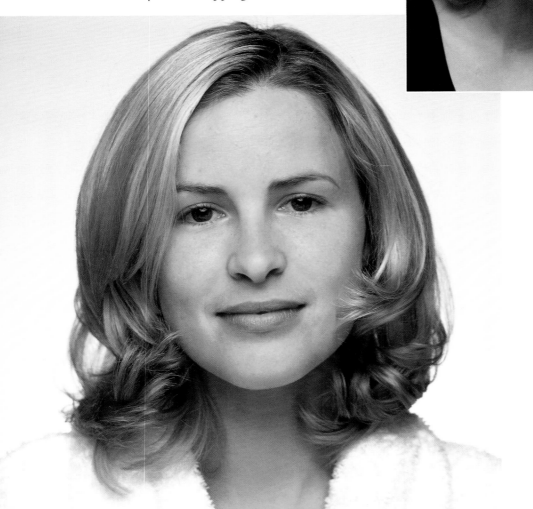

and you are already wearing some, wipe off your make-up at the jawline and test shades there. See which matches your skin tone best and blends closely to your neck. Don't trust the lighting at the counter – you need to go outside into the daylight and check which is best with a mirror.

Whether you choose a cream, powder or liquid foundation will depend on your skin type and how much coverage you need. If your skin seems to absorb foundation, that might be because it's dry, so a cream foundation will be best. Powder foundations are effective in controlling oil build-up on greasier skins. The lightest effect will be from the liquid foundations, which should be applied and spread on with a sponge for minimal coverage.

Be prepared to need two different coloured foundations during the year, especially if you enjoy being outdoors and pick up some colour from the sun. You can mix the two shades together as your tan develops or fades.

Applying foundation

There is no consensus among women or make-up artists about whether fingers or a sponge is better. It comes down to your own preference. In either case, it is advisable to apply a dollop of liquid or cream to the back of your hand, dip in your fingers or sponge and apply from there. If you apply straight from the tube or bottle, you will probably use too much. Less is always more with cosmetics.

Dealing with redness

'High colouring' can result from over-exposure to the elements, from burst capillaries and red veins, or from having frequent flushes. Women with high colouring often feel that nature has overdosed them and that make-up is best avoided because even a little lipstick and eyeshadow can look startling. The answer is light green foundation and moisturizers. The Martian-

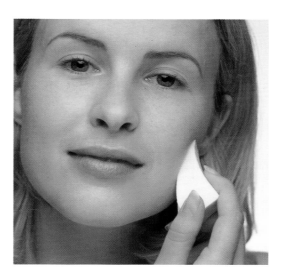

like mint bases neutralize the redness – they work a treat in balancing your high colour so that you can then apply your chosen foundation.

Foundation is good for you

Contrary to what many women think, foundation is good for your skin. I despair when I hear women say that they prefer a 'clean' face to wearing foundation! A good foundation adds protection, along with your moisturizer, from air pollution and harmful UVA/UVB rays. Check what level of sunscreen is provided by a foundation before buying it, and get the best protection for your skin type.

Concealer

For dark circles, lines and the odd spot, concealers are the business. Check out what needs work after you've applied foundation. Your goal is to try to match the skin tone as closely as possible with your concealer (going lighter only results in panda eyes).

Choose a formulation that spreads evenly without being too thin. Use your ring finger to tap the colour over the darkness. Let it settle to see if a touch more is needed. Better to go lightly and then add more than to apply it too thickly initially.

For spots, apply concealer to a cotton bud and dab on directly. Never use the concealer applicator as you'll then grow bacteria in the tube and end up with a face full of spots.

Powder

There is little point in wearing cream or liquid foundation if you don't 'set' it with powder. Foundation will evaporate, get shiny or get on your hands when you touch your face unless you apply a light layer of powder over the top.

Loose powder is the best in the morning. A sponge, puff or cottonwool pad dipped in powder is the best way to press the powder on to the face. Be liberal with the powder as the foundation will absorb much of it in minutes. Any excess can be dusted off with a big brush (which, incidentally, would be useless for applying powder initially to the foundation).

A 'light-diffusing' or 'light-deflecting' powder will make your skin look natural and younger. Heavy matte powders can be

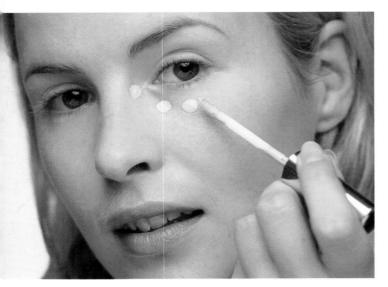

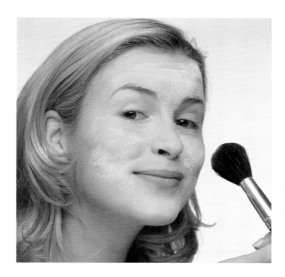

effect you want. If you want the lightest, slightest hint of colour, use a powder blush over your face powder. For deeper colour and to ensure the blush effect lasts for hours, use a cream blush under your face powder and 'top up' with powder blush. A lipstick can double up as a cream blush in emergencies. Gel blushes are popular with the young and the sporty but are too easily smudged beyond their target zones so that you can end up looking like you've had too much to drink!

a bit ageing, particularly on a mature face. Experiment every year or so with a new formulation to be sure your skin's finish is the best it can be.

Evening powder

Try dusting a touch of shimmering powder to the temples, hairline, shoulders and décolletage for devastating effect.

Blush

As with eyeshadow and lipstick, so blush is subject to the vagaries of fashion. But how designers fool around with blush effects for the catwalk should be largely ignored – ferocious red cheeks or a face totally devoid of blush look equally unflattering.

The blush you use depends on the

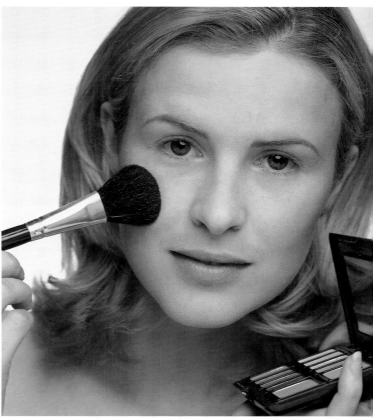

The best blush for you

You need only one everyday blush to work with your whole wardrobe and make you look healthy. You don't want the colour to overpower your eyes or lips.

Never judge the blush colour just by looking at it. As with lipsticks and eye shadows, some formulations are very different between their aspect (what they look like in the display) and their application (what they look like on your skin). Test colours on the inside of your forearm, if you are wearing make-up already.

You need to make two tests to find the right colour. First, the undertone: do you need a warm blush like salmon, terracotta and cinnamon, or a cool blush like rose pink, plum or fuchsia? The right colour will look natural and the wrong one will look, well, wrong. The second test is the strength or intensity of the colour. If you are fair, you want just a hint of colour, the more translucent the better. If you are strong in colouring, with olive or dark skin, you need greater depth and intensity to bring out your striking good looks.

Never choose a blush to go with an outfit. The blush is just a hint of colour to suggest you are in good health or have had the good fortune to have spent a few hours outdoors.

Applying blush

You should aim to apply blusher as if you have just blushed. Hold a smile in front of the mirror. Find the apple of your cheek.

From the middle of your cheek, brush the blush up to the temples, swirling outside the eyebrow. Just a mere hint of blush 'lifts' the face and brings attention to your eyes.

Use upward strokes. Just try applying blush to one side with a downward stroke and the other with an upward stroke to see the difference.

The larger the brush, the softer the effect. If you overdo it, tone down with more translucent powder. If you are in a hurry, soft-coloured blush can double up as an eyeshadow base.

Evening blush

Consider a lighter, brighter blush for the evening, balanced with a deeper blush or bronzer in the hollow of the cheek (as a contour).

Contour powder

If your wide face, chubby cheeks or double chins bug you, then consider using a soft brown blusher or bronzer (the more matte the better) to minimize them. What you don't want is to be Miss Clever Clogs and try to 'reshape' your face with those tricky tips from the beauty columns. Sure, bold stripes of deeper powder are used in photography to great effect. But lighting has a lot to do with the end result. In real life a woman with two brown stripes on her cheeks is just shouting, 'I hate my fat face.'

With contouring, the bushier the brush, the lighter the coverage and the more natural the result.

Eyeshadow

As with your foundation, blusher and lipsticks, there will be one palette of eyeshadow colours that will always be terrific for your eyes and your wardrobe. It's fun to experiment with new colours, formulations and techniques, but most women just want to know what's right for them.

Count up the number of shadows lurking in your make-up bag and on your dressing table. How many do you actually use? Isn't it time to clear out the rubbish? Any over a year old should be binned whether you like them or not because of the likely level of bacteria lurking on the surface. The silly colours you never wear only clutter your morning routine, so chuck them out. Pare down your shadows to just what you need. Read on to find out about your colours.

Your right colours

Color Me Beautiful are experts in getting colours right for women. We know that if cosmetic colours, just like your clothes, are wrong, you will look ill, tired or older. When you have your colours analysed by us, we can give you a palette that will work with your whole wardrobe.

The right colours are determined by your hair colour, eye colour and skin tone. Together they paint a unique picture of you. If you complement your own colouring, your make-up will look more natural and you will look healthier. However, you can 'push' colours to create dramatic effects. The key is to push them in the right direction for you.

If a woman with grey hair and blue eyes wears peach and brown eyeshadows with a terracotta lipstick because she is wearing a brown dress, she destroys the beauty of her natural colouring. That brown dress will look fabulous against pink and grey eyeshadows and plum lipstick, and she will look both brighter and younger.

Women with more 'neutral' colouring – not very dark or light, not very cool or warm – have the most flexibility in changing their colouring with make-up. But consider the chaos in your make-up bag and the possibility for horror results when you mix up, say, a brown eyeshadow with a hot pink lipstick!

It pays to discover the best colours for you and to get advice on the possible directions for experimentation. The result is that you get maximum use out of your cosmetics and you will always look wonderful.

However, there are certain colours that are invaluable in every eyeshadow collection: they are versatile, they work on every woman and they are always in fashion.

Taupe/cocoa: Soft browns that have a hint of grey or pink. Real redheads with freckled skins are better in warmer browns but everyone else can use soft browns. Go deeper if your eye is strong, lighter if your eye is clear or light.

Greyed green: This is a soft yet deep spruce green that is 'greyed down'. It looks wonderful on every eye colour.

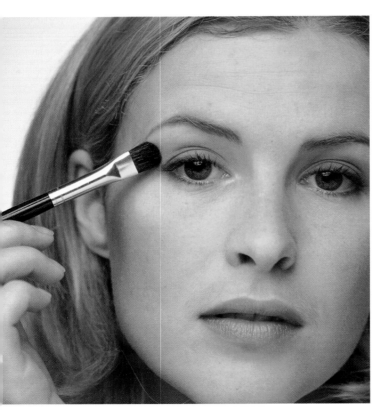

Melon: A warm ivory highlighter that can be dusted over the whole eye as a base or used to highlight the lid or orbital bone. Equally good with grey, brown, navy, pine or plum shadows.

Apricot or pale pink: Warmer-colouring types will glow in peachy apricots while cooler colouring looks fresher in icy, pale pinks. Use as a highlighter.

OTHER COLOUR TIPS

Brown: Hailed by everyone as a must, be wary of the shade on you. The wrong brown can look muddy and make your eyes look droopy and tired.

Grey: Great for smoky effects but requires a very light touch. Wonderful warmed up against a soft yellow or apricot highlighter.

Blue: It's easy to sneer at blue eyeshadow but there are some lovely possibilities. Blue-eyed women should choose grey or teal versions of blue to complement not compete with their irises. On brown and hazel eyes, however, blue is a no-no.

Green: Moss, olive, jade and pine all have possibilities. To make them smokier and more elegant, mix with a bit of grey or taupe. Beware: many greens make blue eyes dull.

Plum: As with other colours, there are many shades, and some create a black-eye effect.

Yellow-based plums are the unnatural ones, while rosier plums or rich purples are terrific on all eyes. Avoid mixing with browns or the eye will look muddy.

Yellows/golds: These tones are quite unnatural so should be limited to mere touches in eyeshadow. Wonderful on golden gals (redheads and strawberry blondes), particularly in the evening.

Pastels: In spring, out come the cotton-candy suggestions for eyeshadow. These are advisable only in teeny-tiny doses in the centre of the lid, just under the brow or in the centre of the lips. Pastel touches look a bit silly during the day except on teenagers, and might be best saved for evening.

Matte or pearlized? Matte shadows vary widely in formulation, with the more matte being quite difficult to apply and blend. Test formulations at the beauty counter using a brush (only the dustiest shadows move with a sponge applicator).

Shiny eyeshadows look luscious in the magazines but ludicrous during the day. Restrict their use to the following conditions: you are under thirty-five and it is after six o'clock in the evening. Limit the placement of shiny shadow to hints in the centre of the lid or just under the orbital bone.

Applying eyeshadow

All remnants of creams, gels or cleansers must be removed in order for the eyeshadow to be applied. If your eyes seem to 'drink up' colour, with your shadow disappearing after a few hours, try using an eyeshadow base cream first. These miracle creams are applied lightly over the lid and orbital bone and are beneficial in three ways: 1) eyeshadow is easier to spread and blend; 2) you end up using less shadow so the product lasts longer; and 3) your shadow won't smudge or develop slicks and will last for hours.

Non-crêpey eyelids can use a light layer of face powder as a base (instead of a base cream). Just dust a bit over the lids when you are doing your face. On older eyes this accentuates creases.

EYESHADOW TIPS

✦ Dust a layer of 'foundation shadow' to even out the colouring. Try a pale ivory, apricot or pink. Use a large, rounded shadow brush for best effect. This brush is also key for blending later.

✦ Less is more. It is easier to add more colour than to lessen the impact of a heavy hand. Use an angled make-up sponge as an 'eraser' when you apply too much.

✦ Work from the outside in. Where you place

your eyeshadow initially is the place that will get the most colour.

✦ Place colour with a smaller brush and blend with a larger one.

✦ Use sideways or upwards strokes to 'lift' your eyes. Going too low with shadow creates droopy eyes.

✦ Deep colours 'recede' or make the eye look deeper, while light colours make the eye 'advance', highlighting the part where you

apply it. Look at your own eyes. Use medium to deeper colours to soften bulgy bits, and lighter colours to make the most of limited space or to draw attention to a particular part, such as the centre of the lid.

✦ Eyeshadow under the eye should be limited to setting your pencil. Avoid pencil and eyeshadow here if you have lines or bags under your eyes.

Evening eyes

Keep the lids very light or use a touch of sparkle. Deepen the arch of the orbital bone with a rich brown or grey. In the 'triangle' corner of the outer lid use a deep colour (navy, pine or plum) and blend with brown or grey, sweeping into the arch.

Eyeliner

Eyeliner adds drama to your eyes, making the lashes appear longer and helping to bring attention to your iris. Techniques change but eye pencil is never out of fashion.

Soft kohl pencils are preferable to liquid liners as you will always get a softer effect and be able to correct mistakes more easily. Keep the tips of your pencils sharpened.

EYELINER TIPS

✦ Keep pencils sharpened to get the line where you want it.

✦ Don't outline the eyes entirely unless you want them to look smaller.

✦ On the top lid, line all the way only if your eyes are large; limit to half or a third to 'widen' smaller eyes.

✦ Always 'set' your kohl liner on the top lid with shadow to prevent smudging.

✦ Raise the line very slightly at the outside edge to 'lift' a droopy eye.

✦ Mix different coloured shadows over your line to create different effects.

✦ Only line the lower lid one third or one quarter (from the outside). Omit altogether if you are lined or puffy under the eyes.

✦ Avoid bright or light-coloured liners that will compete with the colour of your iris.

✦ White liner on the inner, lower lid makes the whites of your eyes look brighter and your eyes larger.

✦ Many eyeshadows can be used wet and can double up as an eyeliner. Use a fine brush to apply them.

Mascara

Many women can't hoover, let alone face the world, without mascara. Eyelashes can never be too thick or too long, which is why mascara is such a key step in a perfect makeover.

Manufacturers keep developing new formulations, but many of us are loyal to a favourite that seems to be our right consistency. It is smart to stick to a winner, but you might be missing out on a wonderful new product if you don't experiment from time to time. When testing mascaras, insist on a fresh disposable brush and only use a sample into which others haven't been replacing used wands. Mascaras are the worst breeding grounds for bacteria.

If you are fair, black mascara will look harsh on you. A brown or grey will be more natural. Otherwise, black is effective on everyone else. Coloured mascaras, unless very deep (like navy, pine or plum), are distracting and take away the impact of your iris.

Removing mascara: To avoid panda eyes resulting from mascara residue, try removing mascara by placing a cotton pad under the lower lashes and using a cotton tip soaked in a non-oily removal lotion. Stroke off mascara from the root to the tip

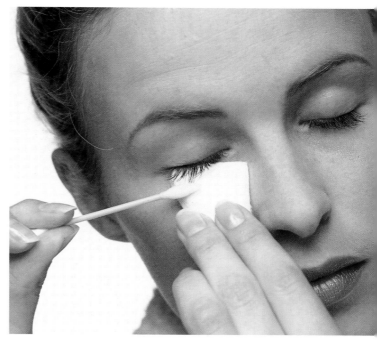

of the lashes using the pad to absorb all the gunk. And presto! Clean lashes and eyes.

MASCARA TIPS

✦ First use an eyelash curler on the lashes to have a wide-awake look. Then apply mascara.

✦ Use mascara on the middle and outside lashes to 'widen' the eye.

✦ Only use on the bottom lashes if you don't have lines or bags under the eye.

- Comb lashes after applying mascara for a more natural look. Do so while they are still moist; if too dry you can damage the lashes.
- Replace mascara every four months to avoid infection.

- Don't pump the brush in the tube: it forces air inside, which dries out the mascara.
- For thicker lashes, powder them lightly before applying mascara.
- Stray blobs of mascara are easier to remove once dry.

Eyebrows

Women cheat their eyebrows more than any other feature. Your brows frame your eyes, so you want to be sure that they are in tip-top shape all the time.

Lucky women with naturally beautiful brows need only give them a quick upwards brush when they finish their make-up. This is best done after getting dressed: pulling a top over your head can brush them down and make you look tired or even angry.

The beauty pundits like to advise us each season on what to do with our brows. One season the brows should be thick and bushy, the next we're told to shave them off and create artificial ones with pencils. If you can remember the natural shape of your brows (or are lucky enough to have retained it), that's the best shape for you. Aside from cleaning up stray hairs or filling in baldy bits, you don't want to do anything else. Trying to create a new look with a pair of tweezers too often ends in tears.

EYEBROW TIPS

- Brush eyebrows upwards and outwards to lift the eye. Stubborn brows benefit from clear mascara.
- Fill in gaps or lengthen brows with a sharpened pencil in a colour that is slightly softer than your natural eyebrow. Never go darker or you'll end up looking like Cleopatra.
- The most natural way to fill in gaps is by dabbing in a soft taupe or cocoa-brown eyeshadow with a short, stubby brush.

- Kohl eyeliners are too soft to use on the eyebrows and will smudge too easily.
- Clean stray hairs from underneath the brows and at the end if they extend in a droopy fashion beyond the eye.
- Keep hairs between brows removed to look well groomed.

The lips

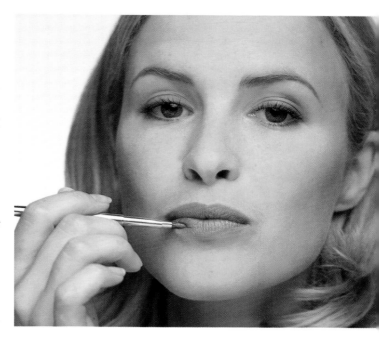

Only the lips compete with the eyes. And many people say that your lips and eyes reveal, in their shape, a lot about you. Big eyes suggest a generous nature and small eyes deceit, they claim; thin-lipped women are mean while their full-lipped sisters are sensuous. What nonsense!

Whatever the natural shape of your lips, you can do plenty to make the most of them. As you've guessed, fuller is deemed more attractive, but with today's tricks even slitty lips like mine can almost double in size.

First, remember that to wear lipstick requires healthy lip tissue. Depending on both your genes and your lifestyle, your lips might need attention before you reach for the red lipstick. Dry lips benefit from weekly exfoliating with your usual facial scrub, a soft toothbrush or a flannel. Wear Vaseline to bed and any time you are just hanging around and don't need lipstick to help prevent the lips from drying out.

Choosing colours

As with your eyeshadows, you need only two or three lipsticks to work with everything. Add to this a lip pencil and gloss, and you have what's required for everything from a game of tennis or a sales meeting to a night on the town.

The three colours every women needs to go with her whole wardrobe as well as her own natural colouring are the right neutral, a pink and a red.

The neutral should be a matte, medium-tone colour such as a terracotta (warm) or plum (cool). You should be able to wear one of these with your entire wardrobe, aside from when you are wearing pink or red, when it is better to match or tone with your lipstick. If you use both warm and cool lipsticks, you and your wardrobe may look rather confused, and it might be time for a professional colour consultation.

Your pink will be warm, such as coral, peach or salmon, or cool, such as rose, cranberry or hot pink. When you wear a pink top, dress, scarf or blouse, tone your lipstick with it. The key is that the undertone should be the same: warm or cool.

Your red takes time to find. All women should have red in their wardrobe to show both confidence and pizzazz. But nothing lets a red jacket, top or outfit down more than a pink or brown lipstick. Your right red will be one of three: a warm orange-red, a cool blue-red, or a true scarlet red.

If red lips scare the life out of you, try using a natural-colour lip pencil first and filling in the lips. Now just add a bit of your red and you will have what's needed to make that outfit, and you, look wonderful.

Lip pencils

The only way to correct uneven lips, to make thin lips look larger or full lips look less so, is with a lip pencil. Pencils provide the added bonus of preventing lipstick from 'bleeding' at the edges, and if you use a pencil to make a base your lipstick will last much much longer.

Always use a sharpened pencil. On thin lips, don't try to create a new lip shape, but follow the outside of your natural lip line to enhance it. On full lips, trace the inner line of the lip edge.

LUSCIOUS LIP TIPS

- ✦ Lighter, shinier shades make the lips look larger; darker, matte lipsticks make the lips look smaller.
- ✦ Pearlized lipsticks will always appear lighter and should be avoided on rough or lined lips.
- ✦ Match your lip pencil and lipstick for truer, more dramatic effect.
- ✦ Use a lip brush for a lighter as well as better application.

- ✦ Try a lip base under your lipstick to help the lipstick hold for longer. Or powder lips between layers of application for a similar effect.
- ✦ Lick the side of a glass or cup before drinking and your lipstick will stay on you, rather than transfer on to the cup.
- ✦ Stick a finger in your mouth and pull out to remove any excess lipstick on the inner lips before it ends up on your teeth.

Evening lips

Wear a deeper-coloured lipstick at night and use a touch of gloss, pastel or shimmering eyeshadow just in the centre of the lips. Try not to get kissed!

Finally, moisturise skin from the outside as well as inside. A light spritz of mineral water over your make-up can give you a dewy freshness if you dislike too matte a finish. Avoid touching your face until the mist evaporates.

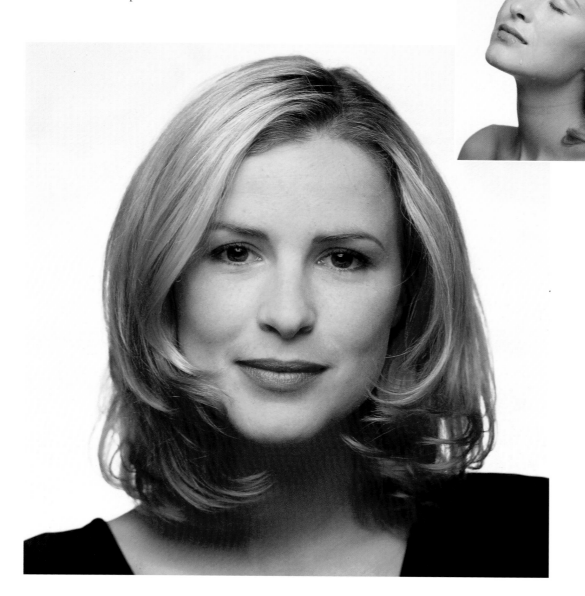

Sun-Kissed
Without the Worry

For years now we have been told about the harmful effects of the sun. The evidence is quite clear: incidence of skin cancer from overexposure to the sun is growing. Even children can develop worrying pre-cancerous cells (skin warts) from being in the sun without protective cream. And to age faster, just expose yourself to the sun without the appropriate sun protection factor (SPF) and watch those lines, sags and age spots form.

But many women love the look of a tan – not that of a leathery buffalo, but a sun-kissed glow that makes them look healthier. Fortunately, there are wonderful cosmetics and tanning creams available today to give you that glowing effect without damaging your skin.

Bronzing powders

Nothing looks worse than dark foundation used to give the impression of a tan. The more natural way to get that glow is to dust a light bronzing powder over your base. The lighter the touch, the better the effect.

Self-tanning creams

Tanning creams have come a long way in the last ten years and are well worth a try if you don't like your winter-white skin with your sundresses. But remember that tanning creams provide no protection from the sun – you must still use the appropriate SPF cream out of doors.

Although you can apply these creams yourself (take your time to do it well), it is good to have someone to help out, especially for difficult-to-reach areas like your back.

TANNING-CREAM TIPS

24 hours in advance: Shave or wax your legs. Test the cream on your thigh overnight to see if you like the colour.

Just before: Brush your whole body with a loofah or special-purpose exfoliating gloves to remove all dry and dead skin. Pay particular attention to joints (knuckles, knees, elbows, etc.) and your back.

Wear old knickers or clothing you don't mind ruining as the cream will stain anything it comes into contact with unless it is cleaned off immediately. Have an old towel handy to sit on until the cream is dry to the touch. Remove all jewellery.

Application: Aim for a thin, even coverage. Wipe away any excess blobs as soon as they are made.

After applying, wipe the palms of your hands clean to avoid unnatural discoloration. But don't forget to do the upper side of hands and fingers that would naturally tan.

Allow the full time (as per instructions) to see the effect before reapplying to deepen the tan. A third application is not advised: the result is not an even deeper tan but dirty-looking skin.

All sun-worshippers should take heed of over exposure to the sun's rays. There is no better living proof of the potential havoc of UVB and UVA rays than studying photos of the young Brigitte Bardot and comparing them to pictures of her now with aged and leathery skin. Many of Bardot's contemporaries who spent less time in the

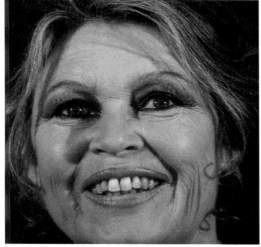

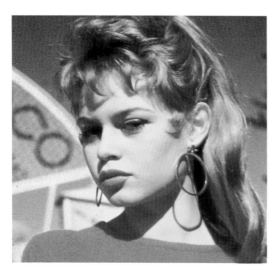

sun look ten to twenty years younger than she. Today skin damage can be made less obvious with dermabrasion or laser treatments that 'burn off' the damaged top layers allowing newer, finer skin to develop. But the process, although effective is expensive and painful. Save yourself the bother by wearing sunscreen all year round.

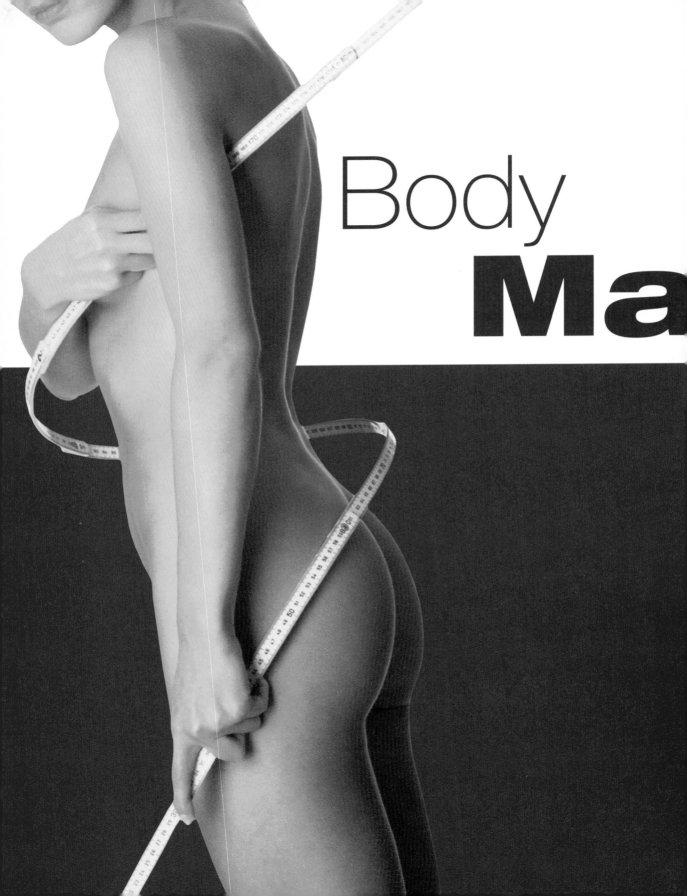

Body
Ma

keover

In deciding what suits you, you are, in many ways, the expert. Over the years, you've had plenty of experience trying different styles, fabrics and designs, and you have a wardrobe full of examples of flattering and unflattering choices.

However, even though you know some safe bets, it can be confusing to experiment and try new looks. That's why it is important to understand the possibilities according to these three indicators: your own Body Shape, Body Proportions and Body Scale.

It's all in the genes

There is both a little and a lot that you can do about your own body shape. First, the genetic prescription: you've inherited some basics like your bone structure, body proportions, height and shape/weight predilection. With exercise and healthy eating you can affect your weight and your shape, but there is nothing to be done about your bone structure, body proportions and height. That is, nothing aside from using clever illusions in the way you dress to achieve what you want.

How you work with your basic body shape – through exercise and diet – will expand the horizon of possibilities. For example, the unfit, pear-shaped woman might feel she cannot ever wear a neatly cut skirt. But the pear-shaped gal who exercises regularly and takes steps to manage the intake of foods that she knows bloats her thighs will have more options. She can look terrific in slimmer cuts of clothes.

Image consultants look at bodies similarly to the way in which doctors and nutritionists do, when they assess how weight is put on and where it is carried. Understanding our hormones and gynaecological endocrinology now seems to be the key to how our metabolism works and to

finding the right approach to exercise and diet. There is no one diet or exercise routine that is right for everyone. The challenge is to understand how you carry weight, what you need to do to keep your metabolic rate working efficiently and how to make the most of your shape.

Your genetic body shape requires its own unique balance of vitamins, minerals, fats, proteins and carbohydrates to stimulate the metabolism effectively. Sure, there are some general principles of healthy eating and nutrition that apply to us all and which are peppered throughout this chapter. But the efficiency of your metabolism – the rate at which you convert food into energy or burn up calories – is the key to maintaining (or losing) weight. For example, a woman who is inclined to retain fluids and can look bloated will benefit from foods, herbs and supplements that drain her lymphatic system and stimulate her circulation. Pear-shaped women are better off eating lightly at breakfast and lunch and enjoying a hearty supper as that is when their metabolism is most active. Women with fairly straight body shapes (i.e. no defined waists and relatively flat bottoms) benefit from eating some protein with each meal as they need to stimulate their adrenal glands to regulate their metabolism.

Hence, if your weight fluctuates or remains stubbornly high despite valiant efforts to eat well and to moderate your intake of fats, processed junk foods and other baddies, resist the latest fad diet promising to help you lose so many pounds in so many weeks because it might not affect your metabolism in the slightest. Instead, find a good nutritionist who will do a proper assessment of your body chemistry and shape before recommending the right eating plan for you. (See the bibliography at the end of the book.)

A New Perspective

MARIE-LOUISE

Marie-Louise's dilemma is one that millions of women understand. Ten, fifteen years ago she had a different body. You know the one: slim, trim and perfectly honed. Those were the days when her life wasn't as crowded as it is today, with a demanding career running a large division of an international PR group, a young family to care for and enjoy, and two households to manage.

She knows that she eats the wrong things at the wrong times and should exercise more. But there are phases of a busy life when doing so can almost seem an indulgence. And, besides, you'd rather coach those young account managers, spend time playing with your kids or enjoy a bottle of wine with your man.

Marie-Louise's basic body shape remains the same – quite straight, with her shoulders and hips about the same and the waist not as distinguishable as it once was. A trimmer version of the Straight Body Shape can wear the structured tailored styles once so successful for Marie-Louise. But once the waist gets broader, these cuts are both uncomfortable and unflattering.

She accepts that her figure now needs a new approach. She has always worn good, quality clothes, but the styles now, although the right sizes, are the wrong cut and fabric.

THE RESULT Today there are many glamorous options that make women bored with boxy, fitted clothes look exciting, slimmer and more modern – not to mention drop-dead gorgeous. These newer 'classics' are less structured in order to suit real bodies living demanding lives.

Marie-Louise could wear this number to the office to influence her team whilst also enchanting her clients, projecting a forward, progressive image.

Take a leaf out of Marie-Louise's makeover experience. Have an image consultant take you out shopping and just try some styles you have never considered. Have the consultant explain how to make the look work for you and how to adapt it to different situations. Marie-Louise bought this terrific outfit and says she feels quite liberated and excited by her transformation.

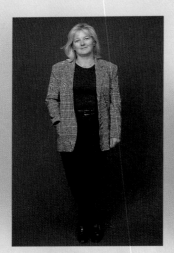

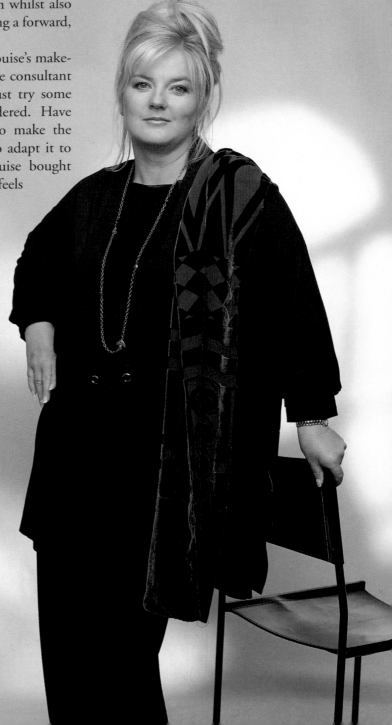

Body Shape

Some doctors define female body shapes according to three types: the ectomorph, who is long and lean; the endomorph, who is curvy and claims to get fat just by 'looking at food'; and the mesomorph, the sporty type who exercises and stays perfect. The followers of Dr Sandra Cabot (author of *The Body-Shaping Diet*) define shape-types by the dominant gland: so the lymphatics are chubby all over; the androids have boyish, athletic figures; the gynecoids are pear-shaped; and the thyroids are the long and lean, with a tendency towards eating disorders.

These medical descriptions can help in our understanding of how and why we put on and retain weight, but they don't help us understand why certain styles of clothes are flattering. That's where we come in. We look at the characteristics of the different female forms and categorize them first of all as Straight or Curvy silhouettes, taking into account the body shape from the front and from the side.

Let's consider your present shape. You might not be your ideal weight or as toned as you would like to be (we'll deal with that in a later chapter), but let's just see if you can determine your silhouette. Stand in front of a mirror and see the outline of your body from the front and side.

Straight

You are a straight type if from the front you see:

- Straight, square shoulders
- No definite waist
- Broad ribs
- Hips narrower or about the same width as shoulders
- Flat (-ish!) thighs

and from the side you see:

- Flat or slightly protruding tummy
- Flat or low bottom
- Little, if any, indentation in the lower back

Curvy

You are a curvy type if from the front you see:

- Rounded shoulders
- Definite waist
- Curved hips
- Round thighs

and from the side you see:

- Indented waist but rounded abdomen
- Curvy bottom
- Definite indentation in the lower back

The Straight Silhouette

You can have a straight silhouette and be underweight, ideal weight or overweight. The important thing is to understand the basics of a straight shape and what to aim for and to avoid in clothes. From there, you fine-tune your look according to your body proportions and body scale, which we will cover later. These are the basics: you will want to take into account your own personality and the latest fashion trends when putting things together. Aim for the cut of your clothes to be simple rather than fussy. Add pizzazz via the colour combinations and accessories rather than choose overly designed styles.

TIPS FOR STRAIGHT SILHOUETTES

Think long tops, neat bottoms, and look for clothes with these qualities:

- Defined shoulders
- No emphasis on the waist
- Minimal darts and gathers
- Tightly woven, neat fabrics
- Pressed-down pleats
- Tailored designs
- Limited texture
- Crisp, defined details
- Classic and man-tailoring

Within the straight silhouette type there are many variations. Looking into a mirror, do you see one of these dominant shapes?

The Lean Column

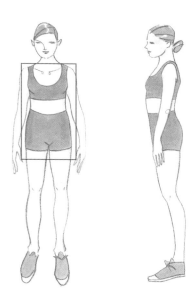

The Inverted Triangle

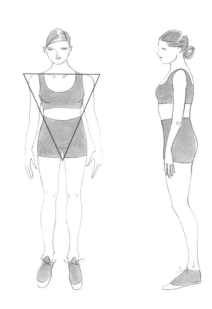

The Rectangle

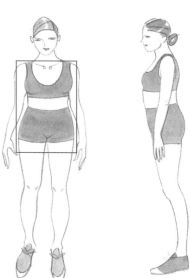

The Apple

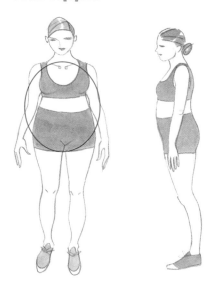

THE LEAN COLUMN

Kate Moss, Twiggy, Liz McColgin

Having a lean, straight body can be wonderful provided you show it off to its best advantage. Figure-hugging designs can look stark – fine if that's the effect you want. You are made for layering, and with layers can make yourself look curvier if you want. To enhance your neat assets, consider a padded bra, and knitted, woven or tight jersey fabrics rather than sheer or fine ones. Sharp, structured jackets will be your best bet. The blazer was made for you.

To accentuate your silhouette for dramatic effect, wear one colour or toning colours head to toe. To achieve the opposite, break up your length by wearing a colour or a pattern on the top half, or try mixing patterns, fabrics or colours throughout.

Beware of cropped tops which can create a 'dotted i' effect. Better if your jackets are not shorter than the hip, and longer still is your most attractive style.

THE INVERTED TRIANGLE

Jamie Lee Curtis, Jennifer Saunders, Brigitte Nielsen

Your broad shoulders will be a terrific asset but when you want to minimize their impact, wear styles with minimal, or zero, padding. Dolman sleeves also help. Very skimpy, slightly too small tops and jackets will only make your shoulders look broader.

Your narrow hips are the envy of us all so make sure we see them. No 'relaxed fit' jeans for you – wear classic or slim-line cuts to show off. Slim trousers and skirts do not mean discomfort. Get the size easy but the silhouette neat to show off what you've got.

If you have a full bust, avoid details (pockets, lapels) on your blouses and jackets in this area. Shorter sleeves are best if they end at the elbow. Going sleeveless is a good option too.

THE RECTANGLE

Zoë Ball, Diane Keaton, Tara Palmer-Tomkinson

Your figure can be as sexy as an hourglass if you wear the right clothes. In addition to the general guidelines above, decide where you want to have the attention then minimize detail everywhere else. If you have great legs, show them to their advantage with flattering skirt lengths, lovely hosiery and super shoes.

If your neck isn't very long and you want attention near your face, remember to open up the neckline: a V-neck works most effectively to draw the eye up. Conversely, if your neck is an asset, see if you can make more of it with a striking necklace or scarf.

If trim but aware that your waistline is wide (no amount of sit-ups will shrink a broad ribcage), wear your belts slung low over the hips (best if your legs are average to long in length).

Jackets that create a slight waist (not cinched, just slight) will be an option, along with the less structured, long, cardigan styles. Watch the buttoning on blazers and jackets. Make sure the key button is not on your widest point (above or below your widest point will be much better).

THE APPLE SHAPE

Roseanne, Dawn French, Ruby Wax

You are carrying a few extra pounds, but you know that underneath lurks a rectangle (dying to get out). Follow the same advice as the other straight bodies – especially about keeping it simple and uncluttered at the waist – but choose softer fabrics for comfort. Soft-gathering or slightly elasticated waists will be a must for you. Choose trousers and skirts in soft fabrics, not stiff ones (such as denim, gabardine and raw silk), and without excessive volume but with the ease where you need it.

If your waistline is approaching your bustline in width, choose loose-fitting tops to avoid showing off a rather matronly 'shelf'. Create the illusion of a longer, leaner top by wearing blouses out (or over) skirts and trousers.

The Curvy Silhouette

Just as with straight bodies, you want to show off what you've got by wearing complementary designs and fabrics. Curves turn into bulk if you wear the wrong things. The wrong cut or the wrong fabric can transform you from lovely to chubby.

Take those curves into account when selecting clothes, but don't let them prevent you from expressing your personality or having fun with the latest fashions. If your body is bugging you and you don't want to draw attention to it, hit the accessories counters and have fun with your shoes, jewellery and scarves. Remember that your face is the centre of communication. If your make-up and hair aren't making the most of your features, we will skip your face and focus on your body. If you want us to appreciate your lovely eyes, skin and smile, then devote your attentions to them while you get your body back into shape.

TIPS FOR CURVY SILHOUETTES

Think soft and easy, and look for clothes with the following qualities:

◆ Easy tailoring

◆ Soft fabrics

◆ Fitted styles that show off your waist

◆ Rounded or set-in shoulders with modest padding

◆ Rounded details, such as shawl collars rather than peaked lapels

◆ Soft gathers and unpressed pleats at the waistline

◆ Narrow trousers that don't hug the legs

◆ Full or tapered skirts in soft fabrics

Just as with the straight silhouette, there are variations within the curved body type. Look into a mirror and see which of these dominant shapes is most like you.

NEAT HOURGLASS

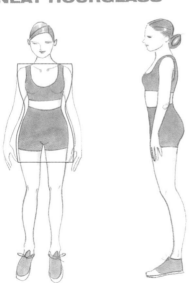

FULL HOURGLASS

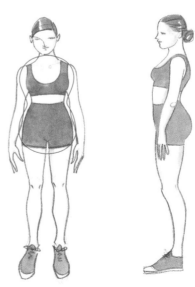

PEAR SHAPE

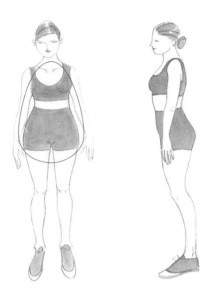

DIAMOND SHAPE

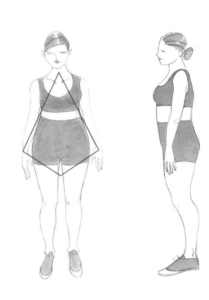

NEAT HOURGLASS/FULL HOURGLASS

**Cindy Crawford, Goldie Hawn, Liz Hurley; Marilyn Monroe, Elizabeth Taylor,
Oprah Winfrey**

There are two versions of the hourglass: one is slim and trim and the other is fuller and more voluptuous. Both want to show off their curves but the neater version will be able to wear more figure-hugging designs than her counterpart.

The Neat Hourglass will be able to wear stiff fabrics (like denim) but will need to ensure that the cut of her clothes isn't too boxy and straight. Her best fabrics will have some 'drape': they will fall gently over the curves rather than stand stiff away from the body. Even though she is trim, she wants ease over the hips and thighs where she is

curved. The cut can be straight but the fabric will need to 'give', so try to have some Lycra, knit or jersey element.

All hourglasses must show off their waist, so dresses and jackets will need definition. If you wear a straight jacket, wear it open with a body or fitted top underneath to provide the definition you need. Stiff cotton, linen or denim tops break down your curves.

The Full Hourglass wants drape, ease and softness in everything. You can wear straight-cut dresses but you will look nicer if the fabric is soft, like silk, jersey or knit, and waisted with a belt (a soft leather, tie or chain belt is better than a stiff leather one with a hard buckle). You'll be lost in bulky cardigans but you will find neat twinsets anything but mumsy on you!

Hunt for the newest cut trousers and jeans that are meant to accommodate a really feminine figure with ample room for the hips and behind. Your jeans can look like denim but should never be denim – denim's too stiff. Instead, try some of the great imitation looks in softer fabrics.

THE PEAR SHAPE

Winona Ryder, Hillary Clinton, Whoopi Goldberg

No amount of exercise or dieting will change the fact that you are built with a smaller upper body than lower body. If you put on weight it is on the hips and thighs, but if you lose weight it tends to go from the torso first!

You have learned several tricks over the years to create the balance you desire in your figure, that is, for the top and bottom halves to look the same size. The way you do this is never to go too tight all over or too fitted on the top. Also, by layering on top or wearing slightly looser jackets and blouses you create the illusion of being fuller there.

On the bottom, due to both your fullness and your curves, you need easy cuts with gathers, vents or darts to accommodate the voluptuous difference between the waist and hips. Tapered skirts or skirts that hang straight will minimize the width on the bottom too. Finally, keep the fabric in your skirts and trousers medium to dark in colour, matte in fabric and devoid of pattern to bring the attention away from that region and to your upper half.

THE DIAMOND SHAPE

Overweight, average to short in stature (and also often shorter in the legs), the Diamond body shape carries her extra weight all over. This is a weight problem that is affecting both your health and your ability to enjoy yourself. Hey, it's no picnic traipsing around stores simply trying to get something to fit. But with a bit of judicial advice, you can look fab while fighting the flab.

It is difficult to generalize about an obese woman, about what shape she would be if she lost weight. Carrying around an excess of sixty or more pounds (that's more than 4 stone, or more than 25 kilos, over what you would ideally be) comprehensively hides what is underneath. You will have to reflect on when you weren't so overweight, or perhaps look at some old photos to discover your basic shape and proportions.

Your objective now is to find clothes that fit and are attractive. As we are still aware of your curves (bust and bottom especially), use soft and drapy fabrics as for all curved types but avoid any waist definition. Long tops and jackets are best on average to tall women. If you are short, jackets that sit on the hips (coordinated or contrasted with the bottom half) will help you look taller.

Avoid black, especially if it is a killer on your complexion. Mid to deep tones will be more slimming, but you need a great colour near your face to keep everyone looking there. Invariably your neck is also full, but don't try to mask the chins under high collars. You will look slimmer if you keep this area open (avoid necklaces). V-necks are your most slimming. Try unbuttoning blouses (two or three buttons) and standing up your collars at the back of your neck while keeping them flat in front for good effect.

Body Proportions

Shape and silhouette are one thing, but then we all have our niggling little quirks that require further advice and fine-tuning.

Pens to the ready, read this list and tick off all the features that apply to you, especially those you consider to be less than ideal.

Long neck	Long waist/torso	Thin thighs
Short neck	Short waist/torso	Full thighs
Thin neck	Narrow waist	Long thigh to knee
Thick neck	Wide/full waist	Short thigh to knee
Wide/broad shoulders	Skinny arms	Long knee to ankle
Narrow/sloping shoulders	Flabby arms	Short knee to ankle
Small bust	Flat bottom	Ugly knees
Full bust	Full bottom	Thick ankles

Necks

Long (and/or thin) neck:

✦ If the length of your neck bothers you, fill in the space by wearing a hairstyle that ends mid-way down your neck. Use chokers, scarves and roll-neck tops to 'shorten' the length.

✦ If your neck is thin as well as long, add 'bulk' by layering, such as a roll neck under a classic collar. Wear a cravat inside your blouses.

✦ Mandarin collars on jackets are particularly good.

Short (and/or thick) neck:

✦ Always wear an open neckline

✦ A V-neck top creates an illusion of a longer, slimmer neck.

✦ Wear a fine chain below the collar bone; longer chains are even more slimming/elongating.

✦ Stand up collars at the back of the neck, and open them low in front.

✦ Oblong scarves tied low are better than squares tied high in the neck area.

✦ Collarless jackets are good but avoid styles that button high.

Shoulders

Wide/broad shoulders:

✦ Softly tailored designs are better than structured jackets with set-in sleeves and defined, padded shoulders.

✦ Jacket piping or trimmed lapels make the shoulders appear narrower.

✦ Raglan sleeves soften the broadness.

✦ V-necks and open collars are better than high buttoning.

✦ For evening wear and swimsuits, the halter neckline is particularly good.

✦ If your neck is long enough, wear choker styles to draw attention inwards.

Narrow/sloping shoulders:

✦ Avoid tight-fitting, skimpy tops.

✦ Layer on the top, for example a loose shirt over a body suit.

✦ Wear shoulder pads with most things. Try various shapes to get the right definition/softness for your overall look. Update the shape of your shoulder pads with changing fashion trends (though not every season).

✦ Horizontal effects create a widening illusion, for example a scarf worn across the shoulders, epaulettes on jackets and dresses, stripes in tops, and wide crew necklines.

✦ Shoulder detail in the form of pleating or gathers is a good idea, for example leg-of-mutton sleeves.

✦ For evening wear and swimsuits, avoid strapless or halter designs in favour of thick straps that angle from the cleavage to the shoulder (that is, the reverse of the halter).

✦ Wear brooches and pins outside lapels.

Busts

Small bust:

✦ Make the most of what you've got with a good bra that creates shape (avoid sports bras in favour of slightly padded styles).

✦ Looser tops will make you appear larger.

✦ Layer on top (T-shirts under shirts then a jacket over).

✦ Wear scarves (neck permitting) inside the neck of your blouses.

✦ Short sleeves 'widen' the bust area.

✦ Use texture and pattern in your blouses and jackets.

✦ Select jackets and blouses with pockets.

✦ Empire waistlines accentuate any bust.

✦ For evening, avoid skimpy fitted styles on top in favour of more substantial fabrics (satin, raw silk) and tailoring.

Full bust:

✦ Open necklines are best.

✦ Use softer fabrics in blouses.

✦ Go for loose not tight-fitting tops.

✦ Look for minimal detailing in blouses and jackets.

✦ Matte and plain fabrics are more elegant.

✦ Necklaces and scarves should end above the fullest point of the bustline.

✦ Avoid very cinched waists.

✦ Soft, tie belts or no belts are best.

✦ A properly fitted bra is essential. Don't hike them too high or let them sag too low.

✦ Avoid layering (which adds bulk), unless in fine fabrics.

✦ For evening, either go sleeveless or wear long sleeves.

Waists

Long waist/torso:

✦ Wear short jackets (if bust allows) or else long jackets with short shirts.

✦ Play up the waist area with belts and detailing.

✦ High-waisted skirts and trousers are great – avoid hipsters.

✦ Use colour and pattern in the top (blouses, jackets) and keep the bottom neutral (skirts, trousers).

✦ Avoid drop-waisted designs in favour of empire styles.

Short waist/torso:

✦ Wear longer-line jackets and blouses.

✦ Have only modest detailing at the waist, such as slightly fitted jackets and dresses; no belts tight at the waist.

✦ Wear thin belts and chains low over hips rather than tight at the waist.

✦ Oblong scarves will 'lengthen' your top.

✦ Layer tops over body suits.

✦ Wear blouses slightly eased out of your waistline.

Narrow waist:

✦ Show it off with belts and fitted designs.

✦ If it is too narrow, layer on top to create more bulk over blouses, sweaters and jackets.

✦ Waistcoats worn open create more width, preventing you from looking too gaunt at the same time as allowing us to peek at your enviable waistline.

Wide/full waist:

✦ If your waist is fuller than your bust or your hips have no emphasis at all at the waist, wear long tops, loose over-blouses and simple, shift dresses.

✦ If you are just broad at the waist, wear thin belts or belts of the same colour as the top.

✦ Or wear belts below the waistline, over the hips.

✦ Single-breasted jackets are more slimming than double-breasted.

✦ Avoid fluffy or shiny fabrics on top.

✦ Oblong scarves will create a slimming illusion in front.

Arms

Skinny arms:

✦ Choose slightly loose but not baggy sleeves.

✦ Wear layered tops, for example bodysuits under shirts.

✦ Textured jackets and bulky sweaters are good.

✦ Short sleeves, blouses and tops with pockets all make you appear fuller.

✦ For the evening, wear blouses and jackets in substantial, not flimsy, fabrics.

Flabby arms:

✦ Set-in sleeves and slightly padded shoulders create balance at the shoulders for full arms.

✦ Avoid tight-fitting sleeves in stretch jersey or Lycra.

✦ Short sleeves should end below the widest point; just above the elbow is flattering.

✦ For evening, sheer sleeves (slightly loose) are great.

✦ When sleeveless, consider draping a stole, wrap or scarf over your shoulders and arms.

Bottoms and Thighs

Flat bottom and thin thighs:

✦ Fitted jackets that flare slightly over the hips (peplums) are good for you.

✦ Shirt or jacket pockets at the hips add welcome bulk.

✦ Dropped waistlines in skirts and gathered styles are both good options.

✦ Team short jackets with short skirts, preferably not matching, for example a plain jacket with a patterned or textured skirt.

✦ Try jackets and tops that belt or tie at the back.

✦ Wear loose waistcoats.

✦ Look for stiff or bulky fabrics in skirts and trousers, such as leather, corduroy, knits, linen.

✦ Pleated skirts suit you.

✦ Wear chunky belts low over the hips; best of all over blouses or sweaters.

✦ Carry a bum bag!

Full bottom and thighs:

✦ Build up the top to balance the bottom. Wear loose-fitting jackets and tops; use layering; and always wear shoulder pads.

✦ Keep the interest on top with colour and texture, and keep the bottom plain, matte and dark.

✦ Avoid stiff or bulky fabrics in shirts or trousers.

✦ Get the fit over thighs, hips and bottom right (namely, easy) and take in the waist if necessary.

✦ Have jackets and tops end above or below the fullest point in the hips.

✦ Gathers in skirts and trousers are necessary but avoid styles that add volume. Minimal gathers over the hips are more slimming than waistlines completely gathered.

✦ Elasticated waists with knife pleating are great in skirts.

✦ Avoid straight or A-line skirts in favour of styles that drape and move (for example cut on the bias, wrap-over, slitted).

✦ Reject turn-ups and trousers or flares in favour of tapered or straight cuts.

✦ Your shortest skirts should end just above or just below the knee. For long styles, go just below mid-calf (tea length) and show a bit of leg.

✦ A slight heel will lift your stature and minimize your bottom.

✦ Avoid very tight jeans or trousers. With stirrups or leggings wear long easy tops.

✦ If you have a nice waist, show it off with fitted jackets and tops. But be careful not to accentuate the hips with very cinched waists.

✦ Control-top tights work wonders but try not to become dependent on restrictive undergarments (like girdles) because they inhibit circulation, make muscles flabby and encourage the build-up of toxins (the dreaded cellulite).

Legs

Long thigh to knee:

✦ Avoid very cropped jackets; hip length or longer is more stunning.

✦ Beware of short skirts and brief shorts: they can make you look scandalous.

✦ Very light or shiny hosiery will accentuate your legs (which might be your objective).

Matte or natural colours will be flattering enough.

Short thigh to knee:

✦ Get skirt lengths to your most flattering point.

✦ Avoid detailing in skirts that 'chop up' the length you have.

◆ Avoid drop waistlines and pockets on hips.
◆ Tone skirt colour with hosiery, even shoes, for best elongating effects.
◆ End tops and jackets at the hip or above the knee (in other words, don't end mid-thigh).
◆ Short jackets with short skirts are best (if your figure allows). Long jackets with short skirts are good; short jackets are needed with long skirts.
◆ Keep interest, colour and details in your tops.

Long knee to ankle:

◆ To exaggerate, wear low-fronted shoes.
◆ Short boots and ankle detailing are good for you.
◆ Rounded or square toes are great. Pointed

tips will elongate the leg further (you might not mind).
◆ Enjoy hem detailing in skirts; gored, A-line and bias cuts are great.

Short knee to ankle:

◆ If your legs are nice, show off what you've got with short skirt lengths.
◆ Minimize the volume in skirts and trousers; neat straight styles are best.
◆ Wear raised heels and open-fronted shoes, avoiding boots or ankle straps.
◆ Tone colour of hosiery with skirt and shoes.
◆ Slit skirts create the illusion of a longer leg.
◆ Palazzo trousers are best if not extreme in width. Avoid flares.

Knees

Ugly knees:

◆ Keep them covered.
◆ Skirts that taper to just below the knee are best.
◆ Mid-tone to dark hosiery is best (matte, not shiny or patterned).

◆ Avoid shorts.
◆ Do calf raises to keep your lower legs toned.
◆ Avoid clumpy shoes and heavy heels in favour of more open-fronted shoes.

Ankles

Thick ankles:

◆ Tone hosiery to skirt colour.
◆ Avoid light-coloured, shiny or patterned hosiery.
◆ Avoid heavy shoes, thick heels, short boots and ankle straps.

◆ Modest heels are better than flimsy or skinny heels.
◆ Long skirts should taper in, not flare out.
◆ Stirrup pants and leggings accentuate your ankles. Opt for slightly fuller styles or classic tailoring in trousers and jeans.

Body Scale

Height and bone structure determine your scale. You might be fine, average or large in scale. If you know your frame is large and you are average to tall in height, opt for:

- a looser fit, particularly on the top half;
- not very fine fabrics (unless you layer them);
- medium to bold prints;
- medium to large accessories;
- longer lengths.

If you know your frame is small and you are average to short/petite in stature, opt for:

- neater fitting clothes;
- fine to medium-weight fabrics;
- minimal volume on the bottom;
- not many colour/pattern breaks from head to toe;
- patterns on the top half if at all;
- average to small accessories.

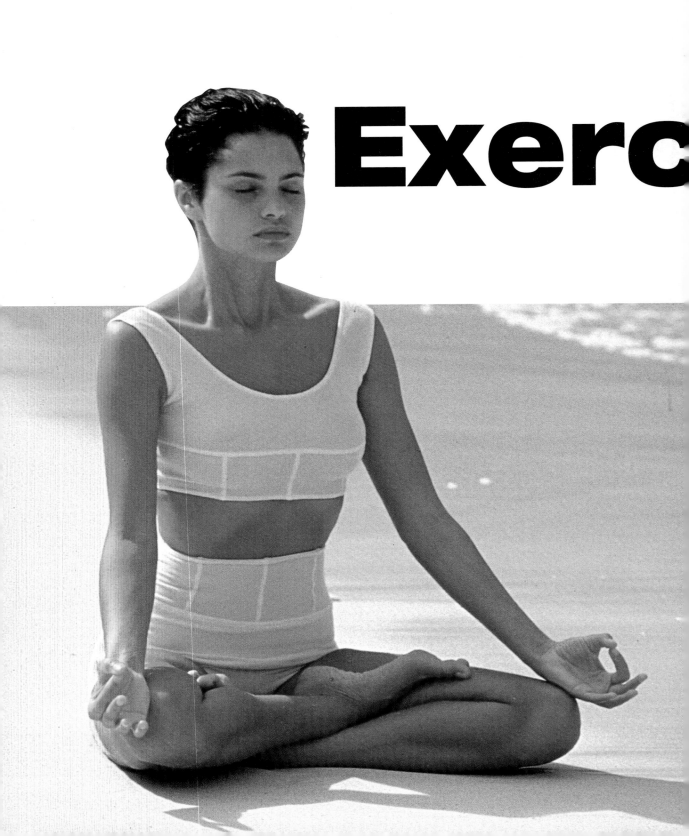

Exerc

se
and Food

Nothing, but nothing, makes you look better than good health and fitness. No matter what size you are, if you eat well and are active you will look younger and more beautiful than your listless chums.

In a matter of only decades, women have changed from being physically active creatures into sedentary lumps. Okay, Okay. 'Not me,' you say. 'I am dashing from pillar to post all day long.' But no doubt that dashing about is in a car rather than walking. In the kitchen and the office you're mainly exercising your fingers (and your brain), while machines bear the load of the physical work.

The sad fact is that over half the women in modern western countries are overweight or obese. Not only is life physically easier on us than it was on our parents and grand-parents, giving us more opportunity to be lazy, but we also eat quite differently now. Our diets are full of fatty, sugary, processed, fake food.

And we are instilling our lifestyle and diet choices into our children. Unless you are a real exception, you opt to drive the kids to school or to their friends in a few minutes rather than spend thirty minutes walking them there. How often do you plan to spend a few hours at the weekends doing an activity *en famille* – a walk in the woods, swimming, a cycling trip? The answer is that families who exercise together regularly are a rarity. Our kids are likely to grow up with the same weight problems as us unless we do something about it now.

What is fitness?

Fitness is not about having cellulite-free thighs or a waist the size of a ten-year-old's. Fitness is having a combination of strength, stamina and suppleness.

Strength: Do you feel rather wimpish when it comes to carrying a suitcase or hauling the shopping from the car? Being able to exert force for pushing, pulling and lifting is how you measure strength.

We need strength daily for small tasks, not just big ones, from opening child-proof caps on bottles and pulling stubborn weeds, to lifting children and taking out the rubbish. If you feel you are asking for more help with basic chores, maybe you need to consider ways to build up your strength. Try doing squats for stronger legs, sit-ups for a tight tummy and a strong back, and arm lifts with weights (bags of sugar will do) for stronger arms. For a stronger grip, squeeze a tennis ball.

Stamina: How often do you collapse in a heap from exhaustion? If climbing stairs or doing errands is starting to wear you out, then it's time to build up your stamina. Build aerobic exercises into your day – walk instead of driving to appointments, for example. Cycling, jogging and swimming also give you the puff you need to be able to dash anywhere in a hurry.

Suppleness: If you are starting to tweak and creak and pull muscles you didn't even know you had, you are probably not as supple as you need to be. You need a flexible body to do the range of little things that come up daily: reaching for that box in the back of the cupboard, bending to get cables into the computer, picking things up from the floor. Try a stretch or yoga class at a gym nearby or get a good videotape of exercises to do at home. You will move more beautifully, develop better posture and look younger as a result.

A New Body
With Exercise

You know the benefits of regular exercise. You look and feel great while improving your heart rate, building stamina and strength, increasing flexibility, developing muscle tone and fitting into your clothes. Your basic body shape won't change with exercise but you can make the most of your proportions by exercising regularly. Buying the exercise tapes or joining the gym is the easy bit. Hanging in there – year round – is the challenge.

We are bombarded all the time with new routines and gear to keep us interested and to lure new recruits to the cause. The key is to find out what you enjoy but also to add variety so that you don't go off it all and give up.

Step 1: GET AEROBIC
Activities such as brisk walking, jogging, swimming, aerobic classes and cycling are the ones most beneficial to the heart, to weight control and to stamina. Commit to doing at least one of these consistently for 20 to 30 minutes three or four times a week and you will be a fit specimen for life.

Step 2: CROSS-TRAIN
Recent research in America suggests that doing too much exercise, especially the wrong kind for your shape, and overdoing it on exercise machines will make you larger and add unwanted inches to your frame. Always get instruction before using any equipment and keep the weight or pressure minimal to avoid building up excess bulk. The correct (for you) use of exercise equipment can help to tone muscle groups aerobic exercises can't reach and you can see results very quickly.

To ensure that you are strengthening your whole body rather than overtaxing certain muscle groups and joints, consider cross-training. This simply means doing a variety of aerobic and anaerobic exercises to get the best balance. Join a circuit-training class – great fun even for the novice – which is done in a gym under the watchful eye and coaxing of an instructor. You are challenged to do a variety of exercises and to use weights in sets. Varying the work rate allows you to catch your breath or gaze in admiration or mirth at the real maniacs.

Circuit training at home is also possible and you need only a skipping rope and a tape/CD player. Pump up the music and skip for one song, then do sit-ups for another, press-ups for a third, then stretch out and repeat. This circuit can take 15 minutes and be repeated for an excellent twice-weekly workout.

STEP 3: ALIGN MIND AND BODY

Exercise can relieve stress but it can add to it too if you don't build in time to recover and reward yourself. Exercise should benefit the psyche as well as the physique.

Yoga is one of the best disciplines for getting the mind and body linked as well as toned. Don't expect to inspire yourself initially by getting a book and trying to follow some exercise illustrations. It is best to find a qualified instructor or a good tape to get initiated in the discipline. You can accept or reject the spiritual concepts while still benefiting from the therapeutic effects of the exercises and the relaxation elements.

T'ai chi helps the even less coordinated develop ease and grace through exercises focused on controlled movements which enhance relaxation. Practice outdoors is key to the discipline. The Chinese have been using T'ai chi for generations and its rejuvenating benefits are now being widely practised by non-Chinese all over the world.

Step 4: KEEP MOVIN'

Be prepared for – no, jump at any chance to try – something new that gets you moving. Every sort of dance is experiencing a revival now, from '70s line dancing, to tap, salsa and belly dancing. When was the last time you came home buzzing from a fun night on the dance floor? The cardiovascular benefit is equivalent to a brisk walk and dancing provides a good workout for the lower body muscles.

Be playful – with kids, dogs – whenever the opportunity presents itself. Even a good wrestle with your partner enhances flexibility and can lead to a welcome aerobic workout!

Jogging keeps you young

Joggers are given pretty short shrift these days. All that panting and pounding of the pavement brings out the worst in many observers. But for those of us who have discovered running as a marvellous way to keep fit, there is increasing proof of its benefits to mind, body and soul. Research from the University of Manchester confirms that jogging keeps your brain as well as your body in shape. Studies testing superfit 45- to 70-year-olds showed that after exercise these characters had razor-sharp mental skills. Pumping blood through the system does more good for the brain than sitting around doing crossword puzzles.

Most joggers and runners confirm that they keep at it mainly because it makes them feel so good, not necessarily just to maintain their weight or fitness. The buzz you feel after a run of twenty to thirty minutes, thanks to all those endorphins pumping through your system, is equivalent to (on some days better than!) sex. And any problem bugging you before a run just isn't an issue afterwards.

If you can walk, you can jog. Just be sure your doctor agrees that upping your daily pace is okay in your current state of health and fitness. Start by jogging gently for three to five minutes, then walking until you catch your breath. Expect the lungs to take a few weeks to get adjusted to the aerobic workout of jogging. Aim to increase your time and not worry about distance initially. There is little benefit in jogging once a week but plenty in doing so three or more days each week.

All that's required for jogging is a good pair of running shoes (not any old trainers) which are flexible yet provide plenty of support. Buy them from a specialist sports store and start by trying a pair at least half a size larger than your normal shoes.

Try running different routes to prevent boredom, or find a chum to join you. Many areas have running clubs that welcome new joggers and can provide lots of advice on getting better. Listening to music is a great way to give rhythm to your stride, but be sure you can still hear traffic for safety.

And if you need any further convincing of the benefits of running, here's the best: you can eat anything you like and maintain your weight if you keep running!

Just exercise more
and eat better

It's that simple. There is little need for weighing food or worrying about which foods you eat together if you just a) watch the volume and type of foods you consume and b) get moving.

Forget calories and focus on food value. You want food to be pleasurable but also to do you some good. If you are in doubt about the value of a food item, don't put it near your mouth. You are not a human dustbin.

Healthy Eating
for Every Body Shape

What you eat and drink, coupled with your exercise routine, affects your body condition. Regardless of your basic shape, your proportions and your scale, you will look your best when you take care of your body from within as well as from without, and learn to view food and drink as fuel for your health and beauty. Try abiding by these eight essential rules for good health, an alert mind and a beautiful body.

The Eight Essentials

1. Eat five portions of fresh fruit and/or vegetables a day. This will get you the essential nutrients (vitamins and minerals) you need to keep fit, keep cool and fight disease. Plus the fibre from the freshies helps you clear out waste and absorb the benefits from other foods.

Don't question this one: just keep the refrigerator and fruit bowl stocked. Either eat them as snacks or discipline yourself to eating one meal a day of just veggies or fruit. Easy peasy.

2. Drink at least 1 litre of water a day. Water is beneficial to your health and to your looks. It flushes the system of toxins and waste by preventing constipation, and it therefore helps protect against bowel cancer too. Plus, water moisturizes the skin from the inside out. You can cut down on expensive creams by upping your intake of water. Guzzle your litres for a week and you'll see the difference in your skin. You'll notice it not only on your face but also on your legs!

3. Get fatwise. Fat is essential to your daily diet but we eat far too much, often without even knowing it (it's hidden in lots of processed food, for example). You know the damage it does, including clogging your arteries and cutting your life short. Be aware of when you are adding fat into your diet via cooking, spreads and dressings. We can get what fat we need from lean meat and fish, whole-grain starches and vegetables. Limit saturated animal fats (butter, cheese, cream) and opt for vegetable oils in cooking such as olive, sunflower, linseed, soya and hazelnut.

    However, fat restrictions taken to extremes will jeopardize your health and beauty. If you have gone overboard with 'fat-freeness', ask yourself if your hair is as shiny as it used to be. Is your skin noticeably drier? If so, introduce some natural fats (preferably unsaturated) back into your diet.

4. Stock up on antioxidants. These are the super-vitamins of our age, known to gobble up nasty free radicals (internal pollutants) in our bodies. Free radicals, if left unchecked, can weaken our DNA and cause heart disease and cancer.

    By eating your daily fruit and veg you are getting what you need. But if you are bombarded with added external pollution from smoking, bad air, radiation and stress,

consider a supplement. Beta-carotene in the form of vitamins A, C and E and the mineral selenium, are the prime antioxidants. Red wines (especially young ones) are also a good source of antioxidants, but a glass or two is all you can justify as medicinal!

5. Limit caffeine to the morning and to three cups max. Caffeine is found in coffee, tea and many cola drinks. It makes you jittery, inhibits the flushing out of toxins (allowing cellulite to build up) and causes headaches. Oh, but there's nothing like a cappuccino and a good gossip!

    As with most dietary dangers, it comes down to discipline and learning to enjoy it in moderation. If you haven't discovered the delights of herbal teas (peppermint after a meal, camomile after a hard day and lemon and ginger to cleanse the system any time), why not try them now?

6. Restrict alcohol to four days a week, max. For those of us who love a drink, it is all too easy to find ourselves in the routine of drinking daily. This is when the alcohol can control you, not the other way round. The limit for women is 21 units a week (a small glass of wine being a unit), but women of slight build should aim lower before signs of liver damage set in.

    Like caffeine, alcohol is a toxin, but alcohol is also a source of unwanted, often uncounted, calories. So those sprawling hips or jelly thighs might be down to drink rather than food. Dependency can creep in unwittingly, resulting in mood swings, plunging energy levels and a weaker immune system.

By all means, relax and enjoy a drink. Just keep it in control and detox your system three or four days a week with other beverages.

7. Graze! If you suffer from energy highs and lows or have an irregular system, eating small meals throughout the day will help you to metabolize food more effectively and keep you feeling energized all day long. High-energy natural snacks, such as dried apricots and prunes, bananas, fruit breads (e.g. date and walnut) and oatcakes, are filling and clear the head faster than anything. Even if you have a big night out planned, better eat something beforehand rather than gorging yourself all at once later. Overstuffing your gut means a restless night and days of trying to get back on an even keel.

8. Know your Body Mass Index (BMI) and keep it in check. Your BMI accounts for your weight (in kilos) in relation to your height. See the table below and determine your own BMI. The ideal index is between 20 and 25. Below 20 could be worryingly underweight and should be watched. If your index is over 35 you need to do something about the excess kilos before you develop serious health problems.

Body Mass Index: A good guide to ideal weight

Body Mass Index	Weight (kg) (to the nearest 1 kg)																				Body Mass Index
45	101	104	107	110	112	115	118	121	124	127	130	133	136	139	143	146	149	152	156	159	45
44	99	102	104	107	110	113	115	118	121	124	127	130	133	136	139	143	146	149	152	156	44
43	97	99	102	105	107	110	113	116	118	121	124	127	130	133	133	139	142	146	149	149	43
42	95	97	100	102	105	108	110	113	116	119	121	124	127	130	130	136	139	142	145	145	42
41	92	95	97	100	102	105	108	110	113	116	119	121	124	127	127	133	136	139	142	142	41
40	90	92	95	97	100	102	105	108	110	113	116	118	121	124	127	130	133	135	138	141	40
39	88	90	93	95	97	100	102	105	108	110	113	115	118	121	124	126	129	132	135	138	39
38	86	88	90	93	95	97	100	102	105	107	110	112	115	118	120	123	126	129	132	134	38
37	83	86	88	90	92	95	97	100	102	104	107	110	112	115	117	120	123	125	128	131	37
36	81	83	85	88	90	92	95	97	99	102	104	107	109	112	114	117	119	122	125	127	36
35	79	81	83	85	87	90	92	94	96	99	101	104	106	108	111	113	116	119	121	124	35
34	77	79	81	83	85	87	89	91	94	96	98	101	103	105	108	110	113	115	118	120	34
33	74	76	78	80	82	85	87	89	91	93	95	98	100	102	105	107	109	112	114	117	33
32	72	74	76	78	80	82	84	86	88	90	93	95	97	99	101	104	106	108	111	113	32
31	70	72	74	75	77	79	81	83	85	88	90	92	94	96	98	100	103	105	107	110	31
30	68	69	71	73	75	77	79	81	83	85	87	89	91	93	95	97	99	102	104	106	30
29	65	67	69	71	72	74	76	78	80	82	84	86	88	90	92	94	96	98	100	103	29
28	63	65	66	68	70	72	74	75	77	79	81	83	85	87	89	91	93	95	97	99	28
27	61	62	64	66	67	69	71	73	74	76	78	80	82	84	86	88	89	91	93	95	27
26	59	60	62	63	65	67	68	70	72	73	75	77	79	81	82	84	86	88	90	92	26
25	56	58	59	61	62	64	66	67	69	71	72	74	76	77	79	81	83	85	87	88	25
24	54	55	57	58	60	61	63	65	66	68	69	71	73	74	76	78	80	81	83	84	24
23	52	53	55	56	57	59	60	62	63	65	67	68	70	71	73	75	76	78	80	80	23
22	50	51	52	54	55	56	58	59	61	62	64	65	67	68	70	71	73	75	76	76	22
21	47	49	50	51	52	54	55	57	58	59	61	62	64	65	67	68	70	71	73	73	21
20	45	46	47	49	50	51	53	54	55	56	58	59	61	62	63	65	66	68	69	69	20
19	43	44	45	46	47	49	50	51	52	54	55	56	58	59	60	62	63	64	66	67	19
18	41	42	43	44	45	46	47	48	50	51	52	53	55	56	57	58	60	61	62	64	18
17	38	39	40	41	42	44	45	46	47	48	49	50	52	53	54	55	56	58	59	60	17
Height m	1.50	1.52	1.54	1.56	1.58	1.60	1.62	1.64	1.66	1.68	1.70	1.72	1.74	1.76	1.78	1.80	1.82	1.84	1.86	1.88	m
Height ft ins	4.11	5.0	5.0½	5.1½	5.2	5.3	5.3¾	5.4½	5.5½	5.6	5.7	5.7¾	5.8½	5.9¼	5.10	5.10¾	5.11¾	6.0½	6.1¼	6.2	ft ins

Guide to Body Mass Index

Fine bones/light frame	Big bones/heavy frame	Comments
15 (less than)	19 (less than)	Worryingly underweight. An eating disorder is likely.
15	20	Underweight. Seek advice of nutritionist.
20	25	Probably ideal.
26	30	Slightly overweight.
31	40	Overweight. Seek advice of nutritionist and increase regular exercise.
35	40+	Excess weight is now dangerous. Seek nutrition/medical attention re. diet and exercise.

Smoking

The harmful effects of smoking are so widely understood and its practice considered so antisocial that it is not included in the list of essential steps for looking and feeling your best. If you have yet to be convinced, put 'Quit Smoking' as your number one priority for a healthier body and more beautiful skin – not to mention longer life.

Good Eating

Avoid adding sugar or eating highly sugared foods as they pile on extra calories, provide no nutrition and wreck your teeth.

Avoid extra, hidden fats by using semi-skimmed or skimmed milk, low-fat spreads and yoghurts. Most biscuits and cakes are loaded with fat. With meat, trim off excess fat and skin. If you love cheeses (so high in saturated fats), have four cheese-free days a week, and on the other days serve yourself a reasonable portion rather than tempt yourself with a lovely cheeseboard to choose from.

Use vegetable oils in cooking (such as olive, sunflower, hazelnut, soya) and soft margarine as a spread (choose one that is high in polyunsaturates).

Eat whole grains, cereals, fruits and vegetables. Unless you are a vegetarian, grill, steam, poach or roast lean cuts of fish, poultry and meat.

Power Foods

Greens: The greener and leafier the veg the better. The chief stars are broccoli, sprouts, cabbage, kale, spinach, cauliflower and turnips. Green vegetables like these contain an anti-cancer agent called sinigrin which protects the digestive system, particularly the colon. Spinach deserves special mention as it is the most effective vegetable in preventing cataracts.

Brazil nuts: A natural source of selenium, which helps to prevent heart disease, cancer and thyroid problems. Selenium is also found in kidneys and oily fish, and can be taken as a supplement. Like most minerals, selenium is toxic if taken in abundance. Limit daily intake to these natural sources or up to 800 units in a supplement.

Berry fruits: All berries are packed with vitamin C but some have additional medicinal benefits. Cranberry juice is a winner for urinary tract infections, especially cystitis. Commercial cranberry juice has a high sugar content (the berries are naturally very sour), so it is best to drink it copiously watered down.

When in season, strawberries should be eaten by the fistful as they contain more vitamin C than any other fruit (by weight). As do cherries, raspberries and gooseberries, strawberries also contain ellagic acid, which gobbles up an enzyme produced by cancer cells.

Tomatoes: Another fruit packed with vitamin C but also being tested as a potential antioxidant in studies with the elderly. Women who eat tomatoes regularly (whole, in sauces, on pizzas) have been proven to be more independent in old age!

Garlic: Any woman with a propensity towards high blood pressure should consider a clove of garlic (or supplement) a day. Studies show that garlic naturally lowers cholesterol levels by up to 10 per cent. Garlic is also a proven winner in warding off colds and infections.

Soy: Thinning bones (osteoporosis) is a worry for all women, particularly as we know we just don't get the amount of calcium we should in our normal diets. By using natural soy sauce or soy curd (tofu), both of which are high in calcium and low in fat, you can strengthen your bones. Soy has also been proven to lower the risk of breast cancer.

Oats: The best low-fat, high-energy breakfast is porridge, which has also been shown to lower the risk of heart disease. Porridge is especially good for insomnia. Just a cupful eaten about an hour before bedtime can ensure a good night's sleep.

You bet . . .
I practise what I preach

What a show-off, I know. But at 47 to still be crossing the finish lines of marathons with a respectable time is no small feat.

I confess to being an exercise junky. No, I am not compulsive, just committed to keeping fit and energized. Weight maintenance spurred me into action in my early twenties but has long since become a lower priority than keeping healthy and spirited. Often it is my PA or a daughter who suggest, when I am particularly ratty, that I 'deserve a run in the park'. In other words, 'go burn off some of that angst woman'. Running 40 to 50 miles a week keeps me sweet as well as trim.

After as little as 20 or 30 minutes of doing anything aerobic, life is in better perspective. If you are lucky enough to be able-bodied you have no excuse not to move. I walk a few miles to and from the office most days and always opt for a bracing dash for 10 or 15 minutes before an important meeting. Gym workouts I don't find as thrilling but do tone those muscles under- or overused by distance running.

As my family has grown, I have worked to build in exercise that we can enjoy together. My girls roller-blade or cycle to accompany me on runs. And we've discovered that orienteering in a wooded forest with a map and compass and conflicting

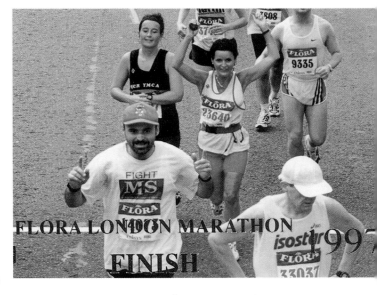

senses of direction is a perfect opportunity to vent frustrations which are brewing with each other. We often end up muddy, in a heap and laughing with each other.

Holidays are never for total 'vegging out' on a beach but always weave in learning a new sport or improving rusty skills with old favourites alongside relaxation. Sporty or outdoor pursuits can create opportunities for meeting new friends of every age and background – a great by-product of keeping fit.

Besides, exercising means never counting calories or fat grams and always saying 'yes' to chocolate.

Your Wardrob
Ma

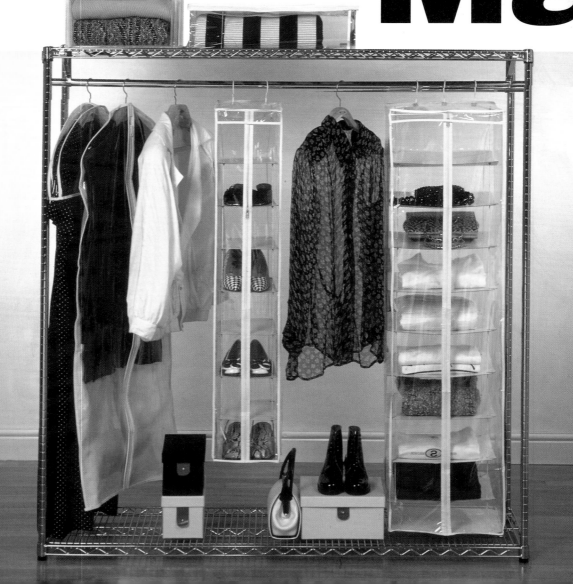

keover

How often have you found yourself wrestling with your wardrobe – fighting to get things in and struggling to get things out because it is too jammed full? You run out of puff looking for that favourite skirt only to realize it's at the dry-cleaners.

All your other skirts are too tight, too tired or just wrong for the jacket and blouse you are standing there in, trying to complete. To finish it all off, you've created a mountain of shoes because you had to dig in the back to locate that perfect pair for today, the first day of spring.

If your wardrobe is getting the better of you, it's high time you got the best from it by Dejunking, Editing, Dividing, Auditing and Restocking. Follow these five steps to mastering your wardrobe and thereby master your life, not to mention your bank account.

Dejunking

Get out the bin liner and, if necessary, a stiff gin and tonic. It's time to sever the umbilical cord formed over the years between you and your gems.

Before you think about tossing out any of your old friends, think of who will benefit from this parting of the ways. The real rubbish items deserve the scissors treatment to ensure that they become dusters and polishers and never, ever, make it back into the wardrobe. Well-worn items that you are no longer in love with will be much appreciated by someone else, so have a bag labelled for a nearby charity shop.

As for disasters – the expensive, hardly worn numbers that will never fit or suit you – they might be recycled and earn you some recompense. Label another bag 'Dress Agency', which can earn you some comfort (namely cash!) for having lost your sanity a few times.

Finally, your real treasures – beautiful clothes that you no longer wear but that you just can't get rid of. These are adding unnecessary clutter to your wardrobe and life. Set aside a nice trunk or old suitcase. Toss in a few mothballs or, better still, cedar balls, and lovingly pack these treasured clothes away. One day you may have a daughter who will find them a hoot, or you may muster the courage finally to toss them out. The key is not to linger about the decision. If you don't wear them any longer, move them out of vision.

Go through everything: clothes, shoes, handbags, scarves, belts, underwear, tights, nightwear – the lot. Leave no corner of the wardrobe or crevice of the cupboard unsorted.

Editing

With the junk out of the way, assess how appropriate the remaining items are for the time of year and your present lifestyle, and then take a critical look at their condition. Work through every single thing.

Seasonal clothes

Anything that you cannot wear in the present season (heavy, woolly winter gear or flimsy little summer stuff) should be packed away (in a labelled bag or two). It is essential to do this twice a year if you want to have a workable wardrobe and not to run the risk of looking out of season.

Check how clean everything is and don't pack anything away dirty. If you want your clothes to last, dry-clean or launder at the end of every season so that they 'rest' without the risk of being attacked by moths or becoming more stale.

Usefulness

If something hasn't proved its usefulness by now, it is unlikely to, so designate it either to give away or sell. You only want to keep items that make sense your present life. If you are convinced of an item's intermittent or future usefulness, decide what is the best alternative location to the wardrobe for it.

Wearability

Any items with stains (that have not yet come out and therefore never will) have no place in your wardrobe.

Do the whiff test on all your jackets, blouses and knits to ensure that they are clean enough to wear to meet royalty, a prospective employer or your mother-in-law. If in doubt, set aside for dry-cleaning or laundering.

Have a good look at what needs repairing. It is so annoying to want to wear something and then to discover that the hem is trailing or a button is missing. Discipline yourself never to put things away until they are repaired. Leave the item out, somewhere annoying like the middle of the kitchen table, and you are sure to do something about it soon.

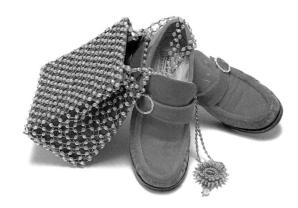

Dividing

Hang everything by categories: shirts together, trousers, dresses, and so on. Then organize by colour, with the plains at one end and patterns at the other. Skirts you might like to arrange in lengths. For trousers, try having the tailored office ones together, followed by the casual ones. Find what works for you, and always arrange hangers in the same direction.

Until you discipline yourself always to hang things back in their rightful places, set aside five minutes a week to put things back where they belong.

Organize your shoes by category – for example smart, casual, and sports or activity footwear – and store them on shoe rails or in shoe bags. Try not to put away shoes in need of a polish, a clean or a new heel.

Drawers need organizing too. Use dividers to keep underwear separate from scarves, for example. Don't stuff drawers – items get crushed and lost, and pulling one thing out can empty an entire drawerful on to the bedroom floor.

Wardrobe losers

Dry-cleaning bags don't protect your clothes. They attract dust, prevent fibres from 'breathing', so that they get stale smelling, and can cause white garments to yellow.

Wire hangers given away by dry-cleaners should be given back as they misshape garments. Trousers hung over the bar of a wire hanger crease so badly that they are, or should be, unwearable.

Wardrobe winners

Padded hangers keep your knits, jerseys and silks, especially blouses, tops and dresses, hanging beautifully in the wardrobe.

Full, shaped wooden hangers provide the best base for jackets and coats.

Skirt and trouser hangers are made for the job, so that these clothes are ready for you when you are ready for them.

Keep shoes on view on rails or in shoe bags to make your choice within seconds. Stacking shoes in boxes means you won't get the full wear out of them because you forget what they look like. Using shoe trees ensures you get your money's worth out of every pair.

Auditing

With the wardrobe dejunked, edited and divided, you can now see the gaps and where you need to replenish items. The best way to go shopping is with a hit list either of essential items or of link items that will revitalize your existing clothes or make things work better together. Have a pen and paper to hand, and go through your slimmed-down wardrobe.

Colour check

How much flexibility do you have with the current colours in your wardrobe? Is your wardrobe all of one shade and in need of a shot in the arm to come alive?

Neutrals

Do you have enough basics (white, black, navy, grey, brown, camel, taupe, stone, beige) in your skirts and trousers, which can be brightened up with other shades?

Neutrals do not always mix with each other. They are most dramatic if worn monochromatically but with a flash of colour or a dash of personality in a print (such as a scarf or blouse).

Brights

Too many or not enough? Or the wrong ones for you? If your neutrals are in pretty good shape, note what new colours (that are flattering on you, of course) you want to get.

Patterns and fabrics

How versatile is your collection? If it is all plain colours and similar fabrics, then you are wearing a uniform. Consider new textures to update your look – a leather skirt or a mohair jumper could be teamed with existing items for work or play.

Style check

I hope that, having read most of this book, you have been able to edit out styles that do not suit your figure. Now, besides noting that you need a new skirt or jacket or whatever, write down what style you are aiming for. If it is a jacket you want, look at the skirts and trousers you already have and make sure it will team with them. Avoid buying something that demands a whole new wardrobe to work with it (unless your budget extends that far).

Links check

The links are the bits that make things work together – a good belt, the right weight and colour of hosiery, well-chosen shoes, and so on. If you compromise on the links, you compromise on the outfit. Which links are missing from your current wardrobe? Is your handbag spoiling your look?

Restocking

Schedule four shops a year into your diary: February, May, September and November. Choose a time in the morning or afternoon (not lunchtime) of a week day when the shops are not crowded and you can get quick service.

THE FEBRUARY SHOP

Shopping just before spring, you will find plenty of fabric options that will be wonderful for many months of the year. Cool wools, jersey and blended knits abound. Now is the time to buy spring and summer suits, as those offered later in the spring are too flimsy for the office (for example, made of linen and thin silks that wrinkle terribly).

Remember to refresh your shoe wardrobe. Clumpy, dark styles that are fine in winter can ruin a lighter look in the spring and summer. Stock up on lighter-weight hosiery and start to restrict opaque tights to really grey days.

Check to see if your raincoat, trench or lighter-weight coat is in good shape to see you through another season. If not, invest in one that is both practical and stylish.

THE MAY SHOP

This is a quick spin through a favourite shop to stock up on essentials like make-up (a different or deeper foundation, a tinted moisturizer, a sheer lipstick or gloss, and sunscreen), tank tops and T-shirts (appropriate for wearing under suits), shift dresses to wear under jackets or 'shackets' (shirts worn as jackets) and a few bits for your holiday.

Before you buy anything for a holiday, audit what you already have and ask yourself how much life is left in it. Don't expect to be able to buy a swimsuit (well, a flattering one!) later than June.

Your handbag or briefcase might be too heavy-looking for the summer months. If so, and if the budget allows, buy a 'lighter' bag to coordinate with your wardrobe neutrals, in camel, taupe or navy.

THE SEPTEMBER SHOP

This is your investment time of year. Audit what you have before you shop and write a list of essential items you need. This should help you avoid the impulse purchases that will gobble up your budget.

Even if you don't travel on business much, imagine that you have to go away for a week and need just a few items to work together in a variety of ways for day and evening. When buying, ask yourself whether the colours, cuts and fabrics are versatile, go together and work with the items you already have.

THE NOVEMBER SHOP

If you weren't convinced of the need for a new mac or a winter coat in September, by now you will be. There will still be plenty on offer but remember not to go too woolly or wintry – unless you live somewhere very frosty, you will only get one or two months' wear from a hearty coat. Macs with zip-out linings are good year-round alternatives and see such hard wear you won't mind replacing them every two years or so.

Buy your heavier-weight tights, gloves, hat (if necessary) and any party gear you might need for the coming festive season. Maybe you can get away with just some sparkling accessories to help transform that all-purpose little black dress. Avoid spending serious money on party frocks that will date or be under-used.

Home shopping

Whether it be by mail-order catalogues, TV or the Internet, working women have many, many services available if getting out to the shops is too difficult to fit in with a busy schedule. (See page 186 for some good mail-order services.)

Beware of the dangers associated with not inspecting the goods yourself, and only buy from reputable sources with easy return policies and refund procedures.

Home shopping can be as compulsive, if not more so, than regular shopping in stores. It is easy to see a bunch of lus-cious shirts or undies in a beautifully shot picture, for example, and order more than you need. If you know that some items on you are particularly tricky, such as shoes, bras or trousers, don't buy sight unseen. Use home shopping for easy items you have confidence in (good brand, have tried before) and it will save you valuable time.

PICTURE CREDITS

4–5, Anita Corbin; 10, Getty Images; 18, 38, 46, Derek Askem; 48, PA News Photo Library; 52, 62, 78, Derek Askem; 102, Images Colour Library; 105r, Rex Features; 105l, Lorraine Felix/Camera Press; 120, Getty Images; 129, Robert Harding Picture Library; 134–135, Ralf Schultheiss/G & J Fotoservice; 145l, The Ronald Grant Archive; 145r, Ginies/Rex Features; 146, The Image Bank; 153, 156–157, Kim Dalziel; 166, Photographers Library; 168–169, Photographers Library; 172–173, Rosenfeld/Anthony Blake Photo Library; 178, Camron Public Relations; 178, Holding Company; 181, Derek Askem.

STOCKIST CREDITS

Julia Alexander *Chapter 2* Pallant
Melissa Ormiston *Chapter 2* Debenhams
Ali Wallace *Chapter 2* Boden and Warehouse
Malcolm Wallace *Chapter 2* Marks & Spencer's
Janice Daley *Chapter 3* Marks & Spencer's
Emma Nicholson *Chapter 3* Jean Muir at Liberty
Rita Ramsey *Chapter 3* Marks & Spencer's
Karen Scott *Chapter 3* Evans
Sutchinda Rangsi Thompson *Chapter 3* Favourbrook
Emma Walmsley *Chapter 3* Dress: Mani; jacket: Debenhams; mango outfit: Jasper Conran
Kate Walmsley *Chapter 3* Blue outfit: Wallis; trouser suit: Jasper Conran
Sue Hoare *Chapter 4* Marks & Spencer's
Julia Rose *Chapter 4* Leather jacket: Warehouse; trousers: Boden; blue jacket: Jasper Conran.
Emily Hutchings *Chapter 5* Marks & Spencer's
Jane Levitz *Chapter 5* White and salmon blouses: Marks & Spencer's
Sarah Wright *Chapter 5* Camel and red outfits: model's own
Marie-Louise Windeler *Chapter 8* Jean Muir at Liberty

UK MAIL-ORDER DIRECTORY

Boden 0181 453 1535
Bras Direct 0990 34 36 38
Bravissimo 0181 742 7085
Cashmere by Design 0171 240 3652
Classic Combination 0800 262 717
Cyrillus 0171 734 6660
Freemans 0345 900 100
Grattan 0345 444 333
Kays 0500 923 923
Kingshill – Diffusion and Designer Collections 01494 890 555
La Redoute 0500 777 777
Long Tall Sally 0181 689 9000
Next Directory 0345 100 500
Racing Green 0345 331 177
Rohan (travel and outdoor clothing) 01908 618 888
Special Collection (disabled fashions) 0800 262 717

Bibliography

Health and fitness

Alexander Technique, Richard Brennan (Element)

Body Foods for Women, Jane Clarke (Weidenfeld & Nicolson)

Boundless Energy, Deepak Chopra (Rider)

Yoga at Work, Miriam Freedman and Janice Hanks (Element)

Food, Susan Powter (Orion)

No-Aging Diet, Benjamine Frank (Dial)

Stop Aging Now, Jean Carper (Thorsons)

Stop the Insanity, Susan Powter (Orion)

The Antioxidant Revolution, Dr Kenneth Cooper

The Body Shaping Diet, Dr Sandra Cabot (Warner Books)

The Busy Body Fitness Manual, Pamela Carsaniga (Allen & Unwin)

The Vitamin Bible, Earl Mindell (Arlington Books)

Ultrahealth, Leslie Kenton (Ebury Press)

Voice

Be Prepared to Speak, Toastmasters International (Kantola Productions)

Never Be Nervous Again, Dorothy Sarnoff (Crown Books)

Powerspeak, Dorothy Leeds (Piatkus Books)

The Sound of your Voice, Dr Carol Fleming (Simon & Schuster)

Your Public Best, Lillian Brown (Newmarket Press)

Beauty

Joseph Corvo's Zone Therapy Pressure Point Massage, Joseph Corvo (Century Hutchinson)

Great Skin for Life, Karen Burke (Hamlyn)

The Art of Beauty, Kevyn Aucoin (Prion)

Colour and style

Bigger Ideas from Color Me Beautiful, Mary Spillane (Piatkus Books)

Chic Simple: Women's Wardrobe, Kim Johnson Gross and Jeff Stone (Thames & Hudson)

The Beauty Bible, Sarah Stacey and Josephine Fairley (Kyle Cathie)

The Complete Style Guide from Color Me Beautiful, Mary Spillane (Piatkus Books)

Image and work

Chic Simple: Work Clothes, Kim Johnson Gross and Jeff Stone (Thames & Hudson)

Presenting Yourself: A Personal Image Guide for Women, Mary Spillane (Piatkus Books)

Total Confidence, Phillipa Davies (Piatkus Books)

Sex appeal

Men are from Mars, Women are from Venus, John Gray (Thorsons)

Sex Appeal: The Art and Science of Sexual Attraction, Kate and Douglas Botting (Boxtree)

The Complete Idiot's Guide to Dating, Dr Judy Kuriansky (Alpha Books)

The Path to Love, Deepak Chopra (Rider)

Index

make the most of yourself with
Color Me Beautiful

PERSONAL CONSULTATIONS AND PRODUCTS

A wide range of services, including Colour Analysis, Style and Make-up consultations, are available through an international network of Image Consultants. Women and men of all ages and backgrounds value the personal advice tailored to meet their needs. Additionally CMB's unique cosmetic system and exclusive scarf collections offer clients simple and elegant means to looking great.

TRAIN AS AN IMAGE CONSULTANT

If you are considering starting your own business and enjoy bringing out the best in others, contact us for details of this rewarding and flexible career. CMB has a vast network of independent Image Consultants who enjoy the support of the leading name in the business.

BUSINESS SEMINARS/ PROMOTIONS AND INCENTIVES

Tailored seminars to ensure staff project the right image are not just entertaining and informative, but make an immediate and lasting impact. CMB can develop exciting sales promotions, incentives and loyalty programmes. Winning makeovers and personal consultations are recognised as a constant draw for both new and existing customers.

For further information, please write to:
CMB IMAGE CONSULTANTS, EUROPE
FREEPOST
London SW8 3BR
Telephone 0845 6033408
Facsimile 0171 627 5680

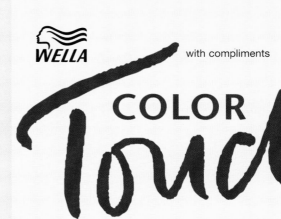

WELLA

with compliments

COLOR Touch

Color Touch from Wella is one of Britain's leading professional, semi-permanent hair colours. With its Shine Intensive Complex – containing award-winning Liquid Hair and Beeswax – Color Touch conditions and strengthens hair giving natural-looking colour with a great shine. If you are having colour for the first time or covering the first sign of grey, Color Touch gradually washes out of your hair leaving it looking beautifully natural.

Now you can try Color Touch FREE (normally worth between £12.50 and £20) with your next pre-booked cut and finish at one of over 4,000 participating, professional hairdressing salons.

How to Claim:
To claim your FREE Color Touch, call the Wella Color Touch Hotline below for details of your nearest salon, then pre-book your appointment with a participating salon. Remember to complete your name and address and salon name and address in the space provided, cut out the voucher and hand your completed voucher to your stylist to qualify.

To find out your nearest participating salon, call the Wella **Color Touch Hotline on tel: 0990 775544**, entering your telephone number including your STD dialling code. The Hotline is open until midnight on 31 December 1998. Calls will be charged at the BT national call rate.

Alternatively, please send an sae marked Color Touch Hotline to: Wella GB, Wella Road, Basingstoke, Hants RG22 4AF and we will send you details of your nearest salon by return.

Offer closes on 31 December 1998.

THIS OFFER IS AVAILABLE ONLY IN THE UK AND NORTHERN IRELAND.

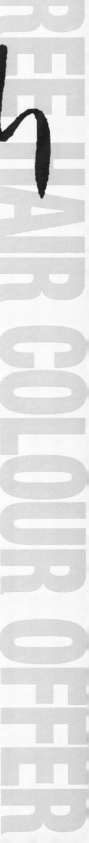

FREE HAIR COLOUR OFFER

Free Color Touch Voucher

About you (Please complete in block capitals)

Your name

Your address

Your phone number

About your salon (Please complete in block capitals)

Salon name

Salon address

Salon phone number

To the customer

When completed, this voucher entitles you to a FREE Wella Color Touch application, providing it is taken at the same time as a cut and finish, which will be charged at full price. Appointments for this offer should be made in advance with participating salons. Only one voucher per person. *Offer open to UK residents aged 18 or over, including Northern Ireland but excluding Southern Ireland. No cash alternative is available and no change will be given. This voucher cannot be used in conjunction with any other offer. Original tokens only. Promoter: Wella GB, Wella Road, Basingstoke, Hants RG22 4AF

Offer closes on 31 December 1998.

☐ Please tick this box if you do not wish to receive further selected mailings from Wella GB.

To the hairdresser

All redeemed vouchers should be handed to your Wella Representative only (no photocopies accepted). You will receive one tube of Color Touch Free in return for every two valid vouchers submitted, delivered with your next minimum Wella order placed. Incomplete or illegible vouchers will not be accepted. Wella GB reserves the right to reject reimbursement of vouchers that it believes not to have been accepted in accordance with its terms.

All vouchers must be submitted by 31 January 1999.

CMB IMAGE CONSULTANTS

CMB Australia
Color Me Beautiful Pty. Ltd.
P.O. Box 329
Kellyville
New South Wales 2155
Australia

Tel. +61 2 9629 2895
Fax. +61 2 9629 5824
Sue Marshall

CMB Canada
105 Mary Street
Pearson Lanes
Whitby
Ontario L1N 2R4
Canada

Tel. +1 905 666 5547
Fax. +1 905 666 8232
Marie Hibbert

CMB New Zealand
Color Me Beautiful (South Pacific) Ltd
P.O. Box 101-435
North Shore Mail Centre
Auckland, New Zealand

Tel. +64 9 441 6474
Jan Sampson

CMB South East Asia
Jill Lowe Int. Pte Ltd
CMB South East Asia
277 Orchard Road
02–39/42 Specialists' Centre
Singapore 238858

Tel. +65 7332016
Fax. +65 7326693
Jill Lowe

CMB USA
Color Me Beautiful Inc.
Dulles Business Park
14000E Thunderbolt Place
Chantilly ,VA 20151
USA

Tel. +1 703 471 6400
Fax. +1 703 471 0127
Steve DiAntonio

CMB Japan
Colormate Inc.
2–10–8 Yagumo Meguroku
Tokyo T152
Japan

Tel. +813 3717 9309
Fax. +813 3725 7070
Yasuko Satoh

CMB South Africa
P.O. Box 6406
Cape Town 7538
South Africa

Tel. +27 21 913 6260
Fax. +27 21 913 6269
Ria Strauss

CMB Ireland
3 Market Court
Bray
Co. Wicklow
Ireland
Tel. +353 1 286 5696
Fax. + 353 1 286 5727
Pat Kelly

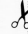